UICC

International Union Against Cancer
Union Internationale Contre le Cancer

TNM
Supplement
2nd Edition

UICC
International Union Against Cancer
Union Internationale Contre le Cancer

TNM Supplement

2nd Edition

A Commentary on Uniform Use

Edited by
Ch. Wittekind
D. E. Henson
R. V. P. Hutter
L. H. Sobin

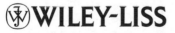
WILEY-LISS

A JOHN WILEY & SONS, INC., PUBLICATION
New York • Chichester • Weinheim • Brisbane • Singapore • Toronto

International Union against Cancer (UICC)
3, rue du Conseil-Général,
CH-1205 Geneva, Switzerland
Fax ++ 41 22 8091810
Email: education@uicc.org
Internet: - http://tnm.uicc.org

Editors:

Dr. med. Ch. Wittekind
Universitätsprofessor für Pathologie
Institut für Pathologie, Universitätsklinikum
Liebigstraße 26
D-04103 LEIPZIG

Dr. D. E. Henson
Clinical Associate Professor of Pathology
Uniformed Services University of the Health Sciences
Bethesda, MD, USA
Cancer Biomarkers Research Group, Division of Cancer Prevention
National Cancer Institute, Bethesda, MD 20892, USA

Dr. R. V. P. Hutter
Clinical Professor of Pathology
University of Medicine and Dentistry
New Jersey Medical School, Newark, NJ
Department of Pathology, Saint Barnabas Medical Center
Old Short Hills Road, Livingston, NJ 07039, USA

Dr. L. H. Sobin
Chief, Division of Gastrointestinal Pathology, Professor of Pathology
Armed Forces Institute of Pathology, Washington, DC 20306, USA
Uniformed Services University of the Health Sciences
Bethesda, MD, USA

Former edition:
ISBN 3-540-56556-6 Springer-Verlag Berlin Heidelberg New York 1993
ISBN 0-387-56556-6 Springer-Verlag New York Berlin Heidelberg 1993

This book is printed on acid-free paper. ⊗

For ordering and customer service, call 1-800-CALL-WILEY.

Library of Congress Cataloging-in-Publication Data:

Library of Congress Cataloging-in-Publication Data is available
0-471-37939-5

Printed in the United States of America.

10 9 8 7 6 5 4 3 2 1

Contents

Preface   XIII
Acknowledgments   XVII
Abbreviations   XIX

Explanatory Notes — General   1

The General Rules of the TNM System   1
The TNM Clinical and Pathological Classifications   4
 T/pT Classification   4
 Regional Lymph Nodes   6
 N/pN Classification   7
  Isolated Tumour Cells   7
 Sentinel Lymph Node   7
 Isolated Tumour Cells   8
 M Classification   8
  Isolated Tumour Cells   8
 Who Is Responsible for TNM Coding?   8
 The Significance of X   9
 Stage Grouping   9
 Residual Tumour (R) Classification   10
 Additional Descriptors   13
 L Classification   14
 V Classification   14
 Recurrent Tumour, r Symbol   14
 Staging of Tumours for Which No TNM Classification is
  Provided   15
 Histopathological Grading   15
References   17

Explanatory Notes–Specific Anatomical Sites   23

Head and Neck Tumours   23
  General   23
    Anatomy   23
    Extension to Adjacent Sites   23
    Adjacent Structures   24
    Regional Lymph Nodes   24
    N Classification   27
  Lip and Oral Cavity   28
    Lip   28
    Oral Cavity   28
  Pharynx   29
    Oropharynx   29
    Nasopharynx   29
    Hypopharynx   30
    Larynx   30
    Anatomical Definitions   31
    Pathological Criteria of Impaired Vocal Cord Mobility or
      Vocal Cord Fixation   31
    Associated Carcinoma In Situ   32
    Paranasal Sinuses   32
    Salivary Glands   32
  Digestive System Tumours   33
    Rules for Classification   33
    Oesophagus   33
    Stomach   34
      T Classification   36
    Small Intestine   36
    Colon and Rectum   36
      Local Recurrence   37
      Regional Lymph Nodes   37
      T/pT Classification   38
      N/pN Classification   39
      M Classification   39
  Anal Canal   39
    Rules for Classification   39
  Liver   39
    Rules for Classification   39
    Regional Lymph Nodes   40
    T/pT Classification   40
  Gallbladder   40
  Extrahepatic Bile Ducts   41
  Ampulla of Vater   41
  Pancreas   41

Lung   42
  Rules for Classification   42
  T Classification   42
  M Classification   43
  Small Cell Carcinoma   43
Bone Tumours   43
Soft Tissue Tumours   44
Skin Tumours   44
  Carcinoma of Skin   44
  Malignant Melanoma of Skin   44
  Breast Tumours   45
  Rules for Classification   45
  Regional Lymph Nodes   46
  T Classification   46
  N/pN Classification   47
Gynaecological Tumours   47
  Vulva   47
  Vagina   48
  Cervix Uteri   48
  Corpus Uteri   49
  Ovary   50
  Fallopian Tube   51
  Gestational Trophoblastic Tumours   51
Urological Tumours   52
  Penis   52
  Prostate   52
  Testis   53
  Kidney   54
  Renal Pelvis and Ureter   55
  Urinary Bladder   55
  Urethra   57
Ophthalmic Tumours   57
  Carcinoma of Eyelid   57
  Carcinoma of Conjunctiva   57
  Malignant Melanoma of Conjunctiva   57
Hodgkin and Non-Hodgkin Lymphomas   57
Appendix   59
References   69

Site-Specific Recommendations for pT and pN   73

Introduction   73
Head and Neck Tumours   74
  pT–Primary Tumour   74

pN–Regional Lymph Nodes 75
Thyroid Gland 77
Digestive System Tumours 77
  pT–Primary Tumour 77
  pN–Regional Lymph Nodes 80
Lung and Pleural Tumours 82
  pT–Primary Tumour 82
  pN–Regional Lymph Nodes 82
Tumours of Bone and Soft Tissues 83
  pT–Primary Tumour 83
  pN–Regional Lymph Nodes 83
Skin Tumours 84
  pT–Primary Tumour 84
  pN–Regional Lymph Nodes 84
Breast Tumours 85
  pT–Primary Tumour 85
  pN–Regional Lymph Nodes 85
Gynaecological Tumours 86
  pT–Primary Tumours 86
  pN–Regional Lymph Nodes 87
Urological Tumours 88
  pT–Primary Tumour 88
  pN–Regional Lymph Nodes 89
Ophthalmic Tumours 92
  pT–Primary Tumour 92
  pN–Regional Lymph Nodes 93
Hodgkin Disease and Non-Hodgkin Lymphomas 93
References 94

New TNM Classifications Recommended for Testing 95

Introduction 95
General 95
  Perineural Invasion 95
Specific 96
  Gastrointestinal Sarcomas 96
  Malignant Thymoma 99
  Cranial and Facial Bones 99
  Cutaneous T-Cell Lymphoma (Excluding Lip, Eyelid, Vulva
  and Penis) 102
  Chronic Myeloid Leukaemia 104
  Primary Liver Carcinoma in Infants and Children 107
  Adrenal Cortical Carcinoma 109

Liver Metastasis of Colorectal Carcinoma   110
Gastrointestinal Malignant Lymphomas   110
References   111

Optional Proposals for Testing New Telescopic Ramifications of TNM   113

All Tumour Sites   113
Fixation of Lymph Nodes   113
Micrometastasis   114
Markers of Residual Tumour   114
Head and Neck Tumours   114
Thyroid Gland   114
T Classification   114
N Classification   114
Digestive System Tumours   115
M Classification   115
Oesophagus   115
T Classification   115
N Classification   115
Stomach   116
T Classification   116
N Classification   116
Colon and Rectum   117
pT Classification   117
Liver   119
T Classification   119
Extrahepatic Bile Ducts   120
T Classification   120
Lung Tumours   121
M Classification   121
Tumours of Bone   121
T Classification   121
Skin Tumours   121
Carcinoma of Skin   121
T Classification   121
Malignant Melanoma of Skin   122
N Classification   122
Stage Grouping   122
Breast Tumours   123
T Classification   123
N Classification   123
M Classification   123

Gynaecological Tumours 123
    Cervix Uteri 123
Urological Tumours 124
    Penis 124
    Prostate 124
    Kidney 125
Ophthalmic Tumours 125
    Retinoblastoma 125
References 125

Frequently Asked Questions 129

General Questions 129
  In Situ Carcinoma 129
  Clinical and Pathological Stage 129
  R Classification 129
  R Classification and Tis 130
  Positive Cytology 130
  T0 and TX 131
  Synchronous Tumours 131
  Single Tumour Cells and Micrometastasis in Lymph Nodes . 131
  Number of Lymph Nodes 132
  Pathological Assessment of Distant Metastasis 132
  Classification of Brain Tumours 132
  Classification of Primary Peritoneal Neoplasms 133
  Pathological vs. Clinical TNM 133
  When in Doubt 133
  Tumour Cells in Lymphatics 134
  Tumour Spillage 134
  Simultaneous Tumours 134
  Direct Spread 134
  Recurrent Tumour 135
  Unknown Primary 135
  AJCC vs. UICC TNM 135
  Sentinel Lymph Node 136
Site-Specific Questions 136
  Larynx 136
  Oesophagus 136
  Colon and Rectum 137
  Pancreas 138
  Lung 139

Breast 139
Corpus Uteri 142
Prostate 142
Kidney 142
Bladder 143
References 143

Preface

The fourth edition of the *TNM Classification* was published in 1987[1] and a revision was published in 1992[2]. It was the result of efforts by all the national TNM Committees towards a worldwide uniform classification. The classification criteria were identical with those in the fourth edition of the *Manual for Staging of Cancer* of the American Joint Committee on Cancer (AJCC).[3] Although the classification has found wide acceptance, some workers have pointed out that individual definitions and rules for staging are not sufficiently detailed. This can lead to inconsistent application of the classification, the antithesis of standardization. This source of differences in interpretation applies not only to the classification of individual organs but also to the general rules of the system, especially to the definitions of the requirements for the pathological classification (pT, pN). These are specified only for carcinoma of the breast; for other sites, reference must be made back to the general rules, which can lead to variable interpretations.

The TNM Project Committee of the UICC has addressed this problem and collected and considered the criticisms and suggestions from the national TNM Committees as well as from cancer registries, oncological associations and individual users. The result was the decision to complement the fourth edition of the *TNM Classification*[1,2,3] with the publication of a *TNM Supplement 1993*[4] containing recommendations for the uniform use of TNM.

In the fifth edition of the TNM classification of 1997[5] most of the tumour sites have remained unchanged from the fourth edition or contain only minor changes. However, some of the changes have

---

[1] UICC (1987) TNM Classification of Malignant Tumours, 4th edn (Hermanek P, Sobin LH, eds). Springer, Berlin Heidelberg New York

[2] UICC (1992) TNM Classification of Malignant Tumours, 4th edn, 2nd revision (Hermanek P, Sobin LH, eds). Springer, Berlin Heidelberg New York

[3] AJCC (1992) Manual for Staging of Cancer, 4th edn (Beahrs OH, Henson DE, Hutter RVP, Kennedy BJ, eds). Lippincott, Philadelphia

[4] UICC (1993) TNM Supplement 1993. A commentary on uniform use, (Hermanek P, Henson DE, Hutter RVP, Sobin LH, eds) Springer, Berlin Heidelberg New York

appeared in the *TNM Supplement 1993* as proposals. The changes and additions reflect new data on prognosis as well as new methods for assessing outcome. The TNM Project Committee of the UICC is aware of the fact that not all proposals for new classifications or ramifications could be transferred in the fifth edition. Therefore, and because explanatory notes, criticisms and questions from all over the world were considered still important, the decision was made to complement the fifth edition with a supplement, too. This second edition includes the greater part of the contents of the first edition plus a number of new items.

In the two chapters of "Explanatory Notes", the definitions of anatomical sites/subsites, regional lymph nodes and T, N and M categories that are generic or ambiguous are defined in a more precise manner. The minimum requirements for the pathological classification of individual tumour sites and entities are described in "Site-Specific Recommendations for pT and pN."

The UICC TNM Prognostic Factors Project Committee has reviewed several recommended changes and amendments for the *TNM Classification*. These are explained in the chapters on "Proposals for New Classifications" and "Optional Proposals for Testing New Telescopic Ramifications". Where data exist to support these recommendations, we have included relevant references; where they do not, the proposals are based on anecdotal experience and/or general considerations. The UICC TNM Prognostic Factors Project Committee is of the opinion that these changes should be tested in the coming years. Consequently, several proposals for modification of the TNM are contained in this *Supplement*. These are based on the principle of ramification, i.e., the T, N and M categories of the fifth edition remain unchanged but optional subdivisions are given within specified categories. By classifying according to these subdivisions one can later compare and determine to what extent a change of the present categories improves the classification with respect to prognostic statements or with a view to the choice of treatment. At the same time, the basic structure of the fifth edition classification remains unchanged.

Furthermore, recommendations are given for the classification of new tumour sites and for entities that have not yet been formally included in the TNM system.

With the development of new techniques in molecular biology, several methods have been described to enhance the accuracy of the *TNM Classification*. The most important and widely used methods are presented.

---

[5] UICC (1997) TNM Classification of Malignant Tumours, 5th edn (Sobin LH, Wittekind Ch. eds). Wiley-Liss, New York

The TNM Prognostic Factors Project Committee receives questions concerning the use of TNM and how to interpret rules in specific situations. The Committee was of the opinion that some of these questions might interest other users of TNM, and they are listed in the last chapter of the *Supplement*.

The present stage grouping as defined in the *TNM Classification of Malignant Tumours*, 5th edition, is generally based on the anatomical extent of disease, as described by T, N and M or pT, pN and pM. For some tumour sites or entities, however, additional factors are included, namely:

Histologic type	Thyroid
Age	Thyroid
Grade	Soft tissue
	Bone
	Prostate
Tumour Markers	Testis
Risk factors	Gestational Trophoblastic Tumours

The TNM Prognostic Factors Project Committee of the UICC and the AJCC recognize that in addition to the anatomical extent of disease, assessed before and during initial treatment, the residual tumour status after treatment, i.e., the R (residual tumour) classification, as well as other nonanatomical factors (e.g., host factors, biochemical markers, DNA analysis, oncogenes, oncogene products) may be important for estimating outcome. These prognostic factors other than TNM and R are currently under investigation; their importance for treatment planning, analysis of treatment and design of future clinical trials will increase. The UICC therefore published a compilation of prognostic factors[5] (a second edition is in preparation[6])

Institutions and physicians interested in the further development of the TNM system are encouraged to test the recommendations for ramification of the existing classifications and those for classification of new tumour sites and entities, as well as methods to enhance the accuracy of TNM over the next years. Publications of both retrospective and prospective studies are desired. The TNM Project Committee would appreciate receiving relevant information and is available for further information and consultation.

---

[5] UICC (1995) Prognostic Factors in Cancer. (Hermanek P, Gospodarowicz MK, Henson DE, Hutter RVP, Sobin LH, eds). Springer, Berlin Heidelberg New York
[6] UICC (2001) Prognostic Factors in Cancer. 2nd ed. (Gospodarowicz MK, Henson DE, Hutter RVP, O'Sullivan B, Sobin LH, Wittekind Ch, eds). Wiley-Liss, New York

The TNM Prognostic Factors Project welcomes comments from TNM users.

International Union Against Cancer (UICC)
3, rue du Conseil-Général
CH-1205 Geneva. Switzerland
Fax ++41 22 8091810
Email: education@uicc.org
Internet: http://tnm.uicc.org

Ch. Wittekind, Leipzig, Germany
D. E. Henson, Bethesda, MD
R. V. P. Hutter, Livingston, NJ
L. H. Sobin, Washington, DC

Acknowledgments

The Editors appreciate the advice and assistance received from the members of the UICC TNM Prognostic Factors Project Committee, the national TNM Committees and the Surveillance, Epidemiology, and End Results (SEER) Program of the National Cancer Institute (USA).

This publication was made possible by grants number HR3/CCH013713-02 and HR3/CCH417470 from the Centers for Disease Control and Prevention (CDC) (USA). Its contents are solely the responsibility of the authors and do not represent the official views of the CDC.

Special thanks go to Prof. Paul Hermanek (Erlangen, Germany) for his ongoing and invaluable help in the preparation of the manuscript.

April G. Fritz, BA, RHIT, CTR, and Carol Hahn Johnson, BS, CTR, Surveillance, Epidemiology, and End Results (SEER)-Program, National Cancer Institute, USA, provided valuable comments.

The International Union Against Cancer (UICC) provided encouragement and support, and its secretariat arranged meetings and facilitated communications.

Abbreviations

AJCC	The American Joint Committee on Cancer
DSK-TNM	TNM Committee of the German-speaking countries (Deutschsprachiges TNM-Komitee)
ECC	Erlangen Cancer Center (Germany)
ERCRC	Erlangen Registry of Colo-Rectal Cancer (Germany)
FIGO	International Federation of Gynaecology and Obstetrics (Fédération Internationale de Gynecologie et d'Obstetrique)
IPSP	The Italian Prognostic System Project
IDS for CRC	International Documentation System for Colorectal Cancer
JJC	The Japanese Joint Committee
SEER	Surveillance, Epidemiology and End Results Program of the National Cancer Institute (USA)
SGCRC	German Study Group on Colo-Rectal Carcinoma
UICC	International Union Against Cancer (Union International contre le Cancer)

Explanatory Notes — General

The General Rules of the TNM System[1,2]

General Rule No. 1

> All cases should be confirmed microscopically. Any cases not so proved must be reported separately.

Microscopically unconfirmed cases can be staged, but should be analyzed separately.

Microscopic confirmation of choriocarcinoma is not required if the hCG is abnormally elevated.

General Rule No. 2

> Two classifications are described for each site, namely:
>
> a) *Clinical classification* (Pretreatment clinical classification), designated **TNM** (or cTNM). This is based on evidence acquired before treatment. Such evidence arises from physical examination, imaging, endoscopy, biopsy, surgical exploration and other relevant examinations.
>
> b) *Pathological classification* (Postsurgical histopathological classification), designated **pTNM.** This is based on the evidence acquired before treatment, supplemented or modified by the additional evidence acquired from surgery and from pathological examination. The pathological assessment of the primary tumour (pT) entails a resection of the primary tumour or biopsy adequate to evaluate the highest pT category. The pathological assessment

[1] UICC (1997) TNM Classification of Malignant Tumours. 5th edn (Sobin LH, Wittekind Ch, eds). Wiley-Liss, New York

[2] AJCC Cancer Staging Manual. 5th ed (1997) (Fleming ID, Cooper JS, Henson DE, Hutter RVP, Kennedy BJ, Murphy GP, O'Sullivan B, Sobin LH, Yarbro JW, eds). Lippincott, Philadelphia

of the regional lymph nodes (pN) entails removal of nodes adequate to vali-
date the absence of regional lymph node metastasis (pN0) and sufficient to
evaluate the highest pN category. The pathological assessment of distant
metastasis (pM) entails microscopic examination.

TNM is a dual system that includes a clinical (pretreatment) and a pathological
(postsurgical histopathological) classification. It is imperative to differentiate
between these classifications because they are based on different methods of
examination and serve different purposes. The clinical classification is designated TNM or cTNM; the pathological, pTNM. When the abbreviation TNM is
used without a prefix, it implies the clinical classification (cTNM). Microscopic
confirmation does not in itself justify the use of pTNM. The requirements for
pathological classification are described on p. 73ff.

Biopsy provides the diagnosis, including histological type and grade. The
clinical assessment of tumour size should not be based on the biopsy.

In general, the cTNM is the basis for the choice of treatment and the pTNM
is the basis for prognostic assessment. In addition, the pTNM may determine
adjuvant treatment. Comparison between cTNM and pTNM can help in evalu-
ating the accuracy of the clinical and imaging methods used to determine the
cTNM. Therefore, it is important to retain the clinical *as well as* the pathological
classification in the medical record.

A tumour is primarily described by the clinical classification before treatment or before the decision not to treat. In addition, a pathological classification
is performed if specific requirements are met (see p. 73ff). Therefore, for an
individual patient there may be a clinical classification, e.g., T2N1M0 and a
pathological classification, e.g., pT2pNXpMX.

General Rule No. 3

After assigning T, N and M and/or pT, pN and pM categories, these may
be grouped into stages. The TNM classification and stage grouping, once
established, must remain unchanged in the medical records. The clinical
stage is essential to select and evaluate therapy, while the pathological stage
provides the most precise data to estimate prognosis and calculate end results.

The rule that the TNM classification, once established, must remain unchanged
in the patient's record applies to the definitive TNM classification determined
just before initiation of treatment or before making the decision not to treat. If,
for instance, the initial classification T2N0M0 is made in one hospital and is
later updated to T2N1M0 after the patient is referred to another center where
special imaging techniques are available, then the latter classification, based on
a special examination, is considered the definitive one.

After two surgical procedures for a single lesion, the pTNM classification should be a composite of the histological examination of the specimens from both operations.

Example. Initial endoscopic polypectomy of a carcinoma of the ascending colon is classified pT1pNXpMX; the subsequent right hemicolectomy contains two lymph nodes with tumour, and a suspicious metastatic focus in the liver, later found to be a haemangioma, is excised — pT0pN1pM0. The definitive pTNM classification consists of the results of both operative specimens — pT1pN1pM0 (stage III).

For final stage grouping clinical and pathological data may be combined when only partial information is available in either the pathological classification or the clinical classification. The example on p. 2 is expressed as pT2cN1cM0 (stage III). For further discussion on the meaning and application of X (e.g. NX, MX) see p. 9.

General Rule No. 4

> If there is doubt concerning the correct T, N or M category to which a particular case should be allotted, then the lower (i.e., less advanced) category should be chosen. This will also be reflected in the stage grouping.

Example. Sonography of the liver: suspicious lesion but no definitive evidence of metastasis — assign M0 (not M1).

If there are different results from different methods, the classification should be based on the most reliable method of assessment.

Example. Colorectal carcinoma, preoperative examination of the liver: sonography, suspicious, but no evidence of metastasis; CT, evidence of metastasis. The results of CT determine the classification — M1. However, if CT were negative, the case would be classified M0.

General Rule No. 5

> In the case of multiple simultaneous tumours in one organ, the tumour with the highest T category should be classified and the multiplicity or the number of tumours should be indicated in parentheses, e.g., T2(m) or T2(5). In simultaneous bilateral cancers of paired organs, each tumour should be classified independently. In tumours of the thyroid, liver, ovary, and fallopian tube, multiplicity is a criterion of T classification.

The following apply to *grossly* recognizable multiple primary simultaneous carcinomas at the same site. They do not apply to one grossly detected tumour associated with multiple separate microscopic foci.

1. Multiple synchronous tumours in one organ may be:
   a) Multiple noninvasive tumours
   b) Multiple invasive tumours
   c) Multiple invasive tumours with associated carcinoma in situ
   d) A single invasive tumour with associated carcinoma in situ
   For (a) the multiplicity should be indicated by the suffix "(m)", e.g. Tis(m).
   For (b) and (c) the tumour with the highest T category is classified and the multiplicity or the number of invasive tumours is indicated in parentheses, e.g., T2(m) or T2(4).
   For (c) and (d) the presence of associated carcinoma in situ may be indicated by the suffix "(is)", e.g., T3(m, is) or T2(3, is) or T2(is).
2. For classification of multiple simultaneous tumours in "one organ", the definitions of one organ listed in Table 1 should be applied. The tumours at these sites with the highest T category should be classified and the multiplicity or the number of tumours should be indicated in parentheses, e.g., T2(m) or T2(5).
   Combining multiple carcinomas of skin should be done only within subsites (C44.1,2, etc). A carcinoma of the skin in subsite C44.3 and a synchronous one in subsite C44.6 and C44.7 should be classified as separate synchronous tumours.
   Examples of sites for separate classification of two tumours are:
   • Oropharynx and hypopharynx
   • Submandibular gland and parotid gland
   • Urinary bladder and urethra (separate tumours)
   • Skin carcinoma of eyelid and neck
   Examples for classification of the tumour with the highest T category and indication of multiplicity (m symbol) or numbers of tumours:
   • Two separate tumours of the hypopharynx
   • Carcinoma of the caecum and the transverse colon
   • Skin carcinoma of the trunk and the arm
   • Carcinoma of renal pelvis and ureter
   • See item No. 1 of M classification (see p. 8)
3. If a new primary cancer is diagnosed within 2 months in the same site this new cancer is considered synchronous (based on criteria used by the SEER Program of the National Cancer Institute, USA).

The TNM Clinical and Pathological Classifications

T/pT Classification

1. When size is a criterion for the T/pT category, it is a measurement of the *invasive* component. If in the breast, for example, there is a large in situ

Table 1. Definition of "one organ" for the classification of multiple simultaneous primary tumours: the listed sites/subsites are considered as "one organ"

	ICD-O Code[a]
Lip	C00.0,1,2,6
Oral cavity	C00.3-5, C02.0-3, C03, C04, C05.0, C06
Oropharynx	C01, C05.1,2, C09, C10.0,2,3
Nasopharynx	C11
Hypopharynx	C12, C13
Larynx	C10.1, C32.0-2
Maxillary sinus	C31.0
Ethmoid sinus	C31.1
Parotid gland	C07
Submandibular (submaxillary gland)	C08.0
Sublingual gland	C08.1
Thyroid[b]	C73
Oesophagus	C15
Stomach	C16
Small intestine	C17
Colon and rectum	C18-C20
Anal canal	C21.1,2
Liver[b]	C22
Gallbladder	C23
Extrahepatic bile ducts	C24.0
Ampulla of Vater	C24.1
Pancreas	C25
Lung	C34
Pleura	C38.4
Bones	C40, C41
Soft tissues, peripheral	C47, C49
Retroperitoneum	C48
Mediastinum	C38.1-3
Skin (subsite(s) only) except eyelid, anal margin, and perianal skin	C44.0,2-4, 6-9
Eyelid	C44.1
Anal margin and perianal skin	C44.5
Breast	C50
Vulva	C51
Vagina	C52
Cervix uteri	C53
Corpus uteri	C54
Ovary[b]	C56
Fallopian tube[b]	C57
Gestational trophoblastic tumours	C58.9
Penis	C60
Prostate	C61
Testis	C62
Scrotum	C63.2
Kidney	C64
Renal pelvis and ureter	C65, C66
Urinary bladder	C67
Urethra	C68.0
Conjunctiva	C69.0
Uvea	C69.3,4
Retina	C69.2
Orbit	C69.6
Lacrimal gland	C69.5

[a] ICD-O Topography code, 3rd edition, 2000, WHO, Geneva
[b] In this organ multiplicity is a criterion of T classification

component (e.g., 4 cm) and a small invasive component (e.g., 0.5 cm), the tumour is coded for the invasive component only, i.e., pT1a.

2. Penetration or *perforation of visceral serosa* is a criterion for the T classification of some tumour sites, e.g., stomach, colon, rectum, gallbladder, lung, ovary. It may be confirmed by histological examination of biopsies or resection specimens or by cytological examination of specimens obtained by scraping the serosa overlying the primary tumour [56].

3. The microscopic presence of *tumour in lymphatic vessels or veins* does not qualify as local spread of tumour as defined by the T classification (except for liver, testis and kidney).

> **Example.** In carcinoma of the uterine cervix, direct invasion beyond the myometrium of the uterine cervix qualifies as parametrial invasion with T2a/b, but not if based only on the discontinuous presence of tumour cells in lymphatics of the parametrium. The L (lymphatic invasion) and V (venous invasion) symbols (*TNM Classification* 1997, p. 12) can be used to record lymphatic and venous involvement.

4. *Direct spread* of tumour into an *adjacent organ*, e.g., to the liver from a gastric primary, is recorded in the T/pT classification and is not considered distant metastasis; in contrast, direct spread of the primary tumour into regional lymph nodes is classified as lymph node metastasis.

5. The very uncommon cases with *direct extension* into an *adjacent organ* or structure not mentioned in the T definitions are classified as the highest T category.

> **Example.** Retroperitoneal soft tissue sarcoma, 5 cm in size with invasion of the ureter: pT2b

6. *Tumour spillage* during surgery is considered a criterion in the T classification of tumours of ovary. For all other tumours, tumour spillage does not affect the TNM classification, stage grouping or R classification.

Regional Lymph Nodes

1. Sometimes a tumour involves *more than one site* or subsite; i.e., contiguous extension to another site or subsite. In this case, the regional lymph nodes are those of the involved sites and subsites.

> **Example.** Carcinoma of the oesophagus involving the upper thoracic portion and the cervical oesophagus: the regional lymph nodes are those for intrathoracic oesophagus, i.e., the mediastinal and perigastric nodes (excluding the coeliac nodes), as well as those for cervical oesophagus, i.e., the cervical nodes.

2. In rare cases, one finds no metastases in the regional lymph nodes, but only in lymph nodes that drain an adjacent organ *directly invaded* by the primary tumour. The lymph nodes of the invaded site are considered as those of the primary site for N classification.

> **Example.** Carcinoma of the sigmoid colon with direct extension into an adjacent small bowel loop: pericolic lymph nodes are tumour-free, but metastases are found in two mesenteric lymph nodes in the vicinity of the invaded small bowel — this is classified as pT4pN1M0 (stage III).

N/pN Classification

1. The clinical category N0 ("no regional lymph node metastasis") includes lymph nodes not clinically suspicious for metastases even if they are palpable or visualized with imaging techniques. The clinical category N1 ("regional lymph node metastasis") is used when there is sufficient clinical evidence, such as firmness, enlargement or imaging changes. The term "adenopathy" is not precise enough to indicate lymph node metastasis.
2. Invasion of lymphatic vessels (tumour cells in endothelium-lined channels, so-called lymphangiosis carcinomatosa or lymphangitic spread) in a *distant* organ is coded as pM1, e.g., lymphangitic spread in the lung from prostatic carcinoma.
3. Cases with **isolated tumour cells** in lymph nodes or at distant sites should be classified as N0 or M0, respectively. The same applies to cases with findings suggestive of tumour cells or their components by nonmorphological techniques such as flow cytometry or DNA analysis.

   A proposal for classification **of isolated tumour cells** has been published [25]. These cases should be analysed separately.

pN0   No regional lymph node metastasis histologically, no examination for isolated tumour cells (ITC)

pN0(i−)   No regional lymph node metastasis histologically, negative morphological findings for ITC

pN0(i+)   No regional lymph node metastasis histologically, positive morphological findings for ITC

pN0(mol−)   No regional lymph node metastasis histologically, negative nonmorphological findings for ITC

pN0(mol|)   No regional lymph node metastasis histologically, positive nonmorphological findings for ITC

Note. This approach is consistent with TNM general rule No. 4.

Sentinel Lymph Node

The sentinel lymph node is the first lymph node to receive lymphatic drainage from a primary tumour. If it contains metastatic tumour, this indicates that other lymph nodes may contain tumour. If it does not contain metastatic tumour, other lymph nodes are not likely to contain tumour. Occasionally, there is more than one sentinel lymph node.

The following designations are applicable when sentinel lymph node assessment is attempted:

pN0 (sn)   No sentinel lymph node metastasis
pN1 (sn)   Sentinel lymph node metastasis

Cases with or examined for **isolated tumour cells** (ITC) in sentinel lymph nodes can be classified as follows:

pN0 (i−)(sn)   No sentinel lymph node metastasis histologically, negative morphological findings for ITC

pN0 (i+)(sn)   No sentinel lymph node metastasis histologically, positive morphological findings for ITC

pN0 (mol−)(sn)   No sentinel lymph node metastasis histologically, negative nonmorphological findings for ITC

pN0 (mol+)(sn)   No sentinel lymph node metastasis histologically, positive nonmorphological findings for ITC

M Classification

1. In tumours of the gastrointestinal tract, multiple tumour foci in the mucosa or submucosa ("skip metastasis") are not considered in the TNM classification and should not be classified as distant metastasis. They should be distinguished from synchronous primary tumours, for example, those with obvious mucosal origin; the synchronous tumours are categorized as multiple primary tumours, e.g., T2(m).
2. Invasion of lymphatic vessels (tumour cells in endothelium-lined channels, so-called lymphangiosis carcinomatosa or lymphangitic spread) in a *distant* organ is coded as pM1, e.g., lymphangitic spread in the lung from prostatic carcinoma.
3. Positive cytology using conventional staining techniques from the peritoneal cavity based on laparoscopy or laparotomy before any other surgical procedure, is classified M1, except for ovarian primary tumours, where it is classified in the T category [27, 37, 38, 55]. Newer data suggest that the worsening of prognosis as indicated by positive lavage cytology may have been overestimated. Thus it seems important to analyze such cases separately. For identification of cases with positive cytology from pleural or peritoneal washings as the sole basis for M1, the addition of "cy+" is recommended, e.g., M1(cy+). In the R classification R1(cy+) may be used [25].
4. **Isolated tumour cells** found in bone marrow with morphological techniques are classified according to the scheme for N, e.g., M0(i+). For nonmorphologic findings "mol" is used in addition to M0, e.g., M0(mol+).

Who Is Responsible for TNM Coding?

Data for TNM are derived from a variety of sources, e.g., the examining physician, the radiologist, the endoscoping gastroenterologist, the operating surgeon and the histopathologist. The final TNM classification and/or stage grouping rest with a designated individual who has access to the most complete data.

The Significance of X

An X classification of an individual component of TNM or pTNM, e.g., TX or pNX, does not necessarily signify inadequate staging. The practical value of staging in the individual situation is to be considered, e.g., in patients with distant metastasis an effort to assess N is without clinical significance. In selected pT1 tumours of the colorectum, pNX may be the result of the correct decision to treat by endoscopic polypectomy or local excision. Also, experience shows that — at least in some sites, e.g., colorectum or anal canal — in T1/pT1 tumours of low grade the frequency of regional lymph node metastasis as well as of distant metastasis is exceptionally rare and therefore no supplementary efforts need be made to assess the N category. The M is assessed clinically, cM0.
(See also item 5 of Stage Grouping p. 10)

Stage Grouping

1. The term "stage" should be used only for combinations of T, N and M or pT, pN and pM categories. The expressions "T stage" and "N stage" should be avoided; it is correct to speak of T categories or N categories.
2. The stage can be determined exclusively according to the clinical classification (TNM), exclusively according to the pathological classification (pTNM) or based on a combination of clinical and pathological findings (e.g., pT, pN and M or pT, N and M or T, N and pM). If available, the pathological classifications are to be used for stage grouping.

Examples
- Pedunculated polyp of sigmoid colon discovered endoscopically, superficial biopsy: tubular adenoma with carcinoma in situ. Endoscopically, no suspicion of invasion. No regional lymph node or distant metastasis. Clinical classification — Tis N0M0, stage 0.
- Endoscopic polypectomy: adenocarcinoma arising in a tubular adenoma invading the superficial stalk, with clear deep stalk. No further treatment. Pathological classification — pT1pNXpMX. Summarizing classification — pT1cN0cM0 or pT1N0M0, stage I. This is justified because experience shows that regional lymph node metastasis and distant metastasis in pT1 are very rare.
- Primary tumour of head and neck. Clinical diagnosis of regional lymph node metastasis by CT, no sign of distant metastasis. Treatment by surgical local excision of the primary tumour and radiotherapy of cervical lymph nodes. Clinical classification — T1N1M0. Pathological classification — pT1pNXpMX. Summarizing classification — pT1cN1cM0 or pT1N1M0, stage III.

3. In the assessment of distant metastases, the entire situation must be considered. If there is only a clinically determined M1 in an organ which could not be microscopically examined, this finding must be taken into consideration, even when there has been a simultaneous pM0 for another organ.

Example. Colon carcinoma with multiple lung metastases (by radiography). Resection of the colon carcinoma because of stenosis — pT3pN2. Simultaneously, also local excision of an area suspicious for metastasis in liver, histologically found to be haemangioma. Final classification pT3pN2M1, stage IV

4. In the definitions of stage groups "any T" includes T0.

| **Example.** | Breast carcinoma | T0N3M0 = Stage IIIB |
| | Malignant melanoma of skin | pT0N1M0 = Stage III |

5. If T or N cannot be determined, stage grouping is possible under the following circumstances:
   - Despite TX/pTX, stage grouping can be undertaken on the basis of N and M or pN and pM findings.

   Example. A firm head of pancreas with a grossly involved peripancreatic lymph node and no signs of distant metastasis at surgery — TXN1M0, stage III.

   - Despite NX/pNX, stage grouping can be undertaken when M/pM classification is possible.

   Example. A carcinoma of the pancreas with liver metastasis T1NXM1, stage IV. Cases with M1 or pM1 are generally classified as stage IV even in cases of T/pTX and N/pNX.

   - Despite NX/pNX, stage grouping is possible when a T category and M0 are provided.

   Example. Carcinoma of the oesophagus with invasion of trachea, regional lymph nodes not assessable, no signs of distant metastasis — T4NXM0, stage III.

   - Cases of Tis (clinical classification based on biopsy) or pTis (pathological classification based on the examination of the resected lesion) are always classified as stage 0, when combined with NX/pNX and MX/pMX, because by definition no metastases can be present.

Residual Tumour (R) Classification

TNM and pTNM describe the anatomical extent of cancer in general without considering treatment. The residual tumour (R) classification deals with tumour status after treatment. It reflects the effects of treatment, influences further therapeutic procedures and is a strong predictor of prognosis. A summary of important references showing the influence of R classification is given below.

Site	*Authors*
Stomach	Hermanek and Wittekind [18, 19, 21], Hermanek 1995 [22]
Colorectum	Hermanek and Wittekind 1994 [18], Hermanek 1995 [22]
Rectum	Hermanek 1997 [23]
Pancreas	Hermanek and Wittekind 1994 [18], Hermanek et al. 1994 [20]
Liver metastasis	Hermanek and Wittekind 1994 [18], Scheele et al. [48]
Lung	Hermanek and Bülzebruck 1998 [24]

In the R classification, not only is local-regional residual tumour to be taken into consideration but also distant residual tumour in the form of remaining distant metastases.

R0 corresponds to clinical remission or resection for cure. It is appropriate for cases in which residual tumour cannot be detected by any diagnostic means. R0 classification, therefore, does not exclude nondetectable residual tumour, which may give rise to tumour recurrence or metastasis during follow-up. R0, in fact, corresponds to *no detectable residual tumour* and may not be identical to cure.

The R classification can be used after surgical treatment alone, after radiotherapy alone, after chemotherapy alone or after multimodal therapy. After nonsurgical treatment, the presence or absence of residual tumour is determined using clinical methods. After surgical treatment, the R classification requires a close cooperation between the surgeon and pathologist in a two-step process illustrated in Figure 1.

Cases with macroscopic residual tumour (R2) may be subdivided according to the certainty of diagnosis into R2a (without microscopic confirmation) and R2b (microscopically confirmed) [9].

In the R0 group there may be M0 cases as well as M1 cases. In the latter, the distant metastasis as well as the primary tumour must be removed completely.

In tumour resection specimens with formal lymphadenectomy the "marginal" lymph node is the one near the resection line that is most distant from the primary tumour. Involvement of such "marginal" or "apical" nodes or of a sentinel node does not influence the R classification.

Difficulties arise in case of removal of the tumour in two or more parts and not "en bloc". Without an exact and reliable topographical orientation, the pathologist cannot make a definitive assessment of the resection line. In these cases, the classification RX (presence of residual tumour cannot be assessed) is appropriate.

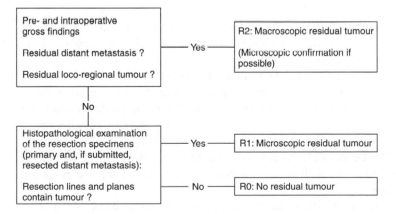

Figure 1. R classification after surgery

The presence of noninvasive carcinoma at the resection margin should be indicated by the suffix (is).

Example. Invasive carcinoma of the breast with associated in situ component. Breast preserving surgery, according to the surgeon, was complete. Histology shows:

a) Invasive carcinoma at the resection margin: R1
b) Invasive carcinoma completely removed; however, associated in situ component at the resection margin: R1(is).

Patients classified for residual tumour by conventional methods and those classified by new specialized methods cannot be compared. To prevent stage migration by refined diagnostic techniques, the methods used for R classification should be stated in the documentation and should be considered in the analysis of treatment results [18].

Examination of resection specimens is done by conventional methods in histopathological processing of areas marked by the surgeon or areas suspicious by gross inspection. Besides these conventional methods, some new techniques have been developed to refine the R classification. Examples of such methods are:

1. Imprint cytology of the resection margin (surface), introduced by Veronesi et al. [54] for breast cancer but applicable to stomach cancer and other tumour types as well.
2. Cytologic examination of ascites or abdominal lavage fluid to detect grossly nonrecognizable metastasis on the peritoneum. This was applied to gastric carcinoma [27, 38, 42]. In the R classification R1(cy+) may be used [25].
3. Examination of bone marrow biopsies in patients without evidence of bone metastasis with monoclonal antibodies against cytokeratin. Such investigations have been described by Schlimok et al. [49] for gastric carcinomas and are reviewed by Pantel et al. [43] (see p. 7 regarding detection of isolated tumour cells and evidence of tumour by non-morphologic methods).

Although there have been proposals (see below) to code a tumour R1 if the tumour is 1 mm from the resection margin, only if the tumour is transected is R1 used, otherwise it is R0.

According to the data from Erlangen (ECC) and Australia, R1 was only diagnosed if tumour was demonstrated at the resection margins (tumour transected). Quirke [45, 46] diagnosed R1 if tumour could be shown 1 mm in distance from resection margin. Compton et al. (2000) [7] also recommended use of the latter definition for the R classification.

The German Documentation system proposes to follow the strict rule, but to record cases with tumour within 1 mm or less from the resection margin separately.

In the R classification the serum level of tumour markers is not considered (see p. 114).

Additional Descriptors

a symbol. The prefix "a" indicates that classification is first determined at autopsy.

On the other hand, tumours which have been clinically diagnosed and classified based on autopsy findings can be classified in two ways:

- Recurrence after a disease-free interval: rpTNM
- Other cases: pTNM

y symbol. Classifying treated tumours.

In the pT classification the extent of cancer before therapy is assessed. After multimodal therapy (neoadjuvant radio- and/or chemotherapy before surgery) this assessment is difficult because of possible tumour regression. Thus such a classification should be identified by the prefix "y" to indicate that this classification has not the same reliability as the pTNM classification after surgery alone. The ypTNM classification as well as the pTNM classification deal with the extent of cancer before therapy. Therefore, ypTNM should consider not only viable tumour cells but also signs of regressed tumour tissue such as scars, fibrotic areas, fibrotic nodules, granulation tissue, mucin lakes, etc. Only in this way are comparisons between patients with and without neoadjuvant therapy in regard to the pretherapeutic tumour status possible.

In all cases with multimodal treatment, information on the extent of histologic regression of tumour tissues should be added. For several sites tumour regression grading systems, mostly semiquantitative, have been published:

Tumour site	Authors
Oesophagus	Japanese Soc Oesopha Dis (1990) [28], Mandard et al. (1994) [35]
Stomach	Jap. Res. Soc. Gastric Cancer (1995) [29, 30], Becker et al. (1997) [3]
Colon and rectum	Dworak et al. (1997) [10]
Anal canal	Klimpfinger et al. (1994) [34]
Pancreas (ductal adenocarcinoma)	Evans et al. (1992)[4]
Lung	Junker et al. (1995) [32]
Lung (small-cell)	Müller et al. (1998) [40]
Lung (nonsmall-cell)	Junker et al. (1997) [33]
Bone tumours/Osteosarcoma	Huvos (1991) [26], Salzer-Kuntschik et al. (1983) [47]
Soft tissue tumours	Schmidt et al. (1993) [50]
Breast	Sinn et al. (1994) [53]

---

[4] Evans DB, Rich TA, Byrd DR et al. Preoperative chemoradiation and pancreaticoduodenectomy for adenocarcinoma of the pancreas. Arch Surg 1992; 127: 1335–1339

L Classification

Lymphatic vessels include those within and at the margins of the primary tumour as well as afferent and efferent lymphatics. Invasion of small lymphatic vessels requires the demonstration of tumour cells (single or groups) within channels that are unequivocally lined with endothelium. If spaces around tumour nests caused by shrinkage during tissue processing cannot be distinguished from lymphatic invasion, L0 is selected (general rule No. 4).

V Classification

For colorectal tumours a tumour nodule in the connective tissue in the lymph drainage area of a primary tumour without histological evidence of residual lymph node in the nodule is classified in the N category as a regional lymph node metastasis if the nodule has the form and smooth contour of a lymph node. However, if the nodule has an irregular contour, it should be classified in the T category and also coded as V1 (microscopic venous invasion) or V2, if it was grossly evident, because there is a strong likelihood that it represents venous invasion [14, 15, 16].

Recurrent Tumour, r Symbol

The prefix "r" is used for classification of recurrent tumours (stage grouping is not appropriate for recurrent tumours). There *must* be a documented disease-free interval. Whereas TNM and pTNM without the prefix "r" always characterize the first manifestation of a tumour, recurrences after curative treatment are described by rTNM or rpTNM. In this way, a chronological TNM/pTNM documentation of the course of disease may be created. An example of such a "pathogram" is demonstrated in Table 2.

For the description of a recurrence in the area of the primary tumour the T categories can be used only in case of recurrence on the anastomotic suture line after partial or total resection of an organ of the gastrointestinal tract.

Example

• Previous total gastrectomy, without remaining local-regional residual tumour.
  Local recurrence at the oesophagojejunostomy involving mucosa, submucosa, muscularis propria and perimuscular tissue - rT3.

In other cases, the recurrence in the area of the primary tumour may be indicated by "rT+".

Example. Local recurrence after simple mastectomy, 2 cm in greatest dimension, with or without invasion of skin or chest wall: rT+.

Table 2. "Pathogram" of a patient with rectal carcinoma

Date	Treatment	TNM/pTNM/R
April 1992	Complete local excision (perianal disc excision)	T1N0M0, pT1pN0pMX/R0
July 1992		
October 1992		
January 1993		rT0N0M0
April 1993		
July 1993		
October 1993		rT1N0M0
	Low anterior resection	rpT2pN1pMX/R0
January 1994		
April 1994		rT0N0M0
July 1994		
October 1994		rT0N0M1 (Liver)
	Liver resection	rT0N0pM1/R0
January 1995		rT0N0M0
Last contact		
January 2000		rT0N0M0

Staging of Tumours for Which No TNM Classification is Provided

Staging according to the rules of the SEER Program [52] is recommended if no TNM classification is provided. Staging is based on the concept of local, regional and distant.

- In situ (noninvasive, intraepithelial)
- Localized (confined to the organ of origin)
- Regional, direct extension
- Regional, lymph nodes
- Regional, direct extension and lymph nodes
- Distant, direct extension or metastasis
- Distant, lymph nodes

These cases should be analyzed separately.

Histopathological Grading

Histopathological grading of tumours of the same histological type is performed to provide some indication of their aggressiveness, which may in turn relate to prognosis or treatment. Grading should follow the recommendations of the WHO International Histological Classification of Tumours.

For most sites, histopathological grading consists of four grades:

G1   Well differentiated
G2   Moderately differentiated

G3   Poorly differentiated
G4   Undifferentiated

In the event that there are different degrees of differentiation in a tumour, one should assign the tumour to the least favourable grade of G1–G4.

Example. Partially well-differentiated, partially moderately differentiated adenocarcinoma of the colon — G2.

G1 and G2 may be grouped together as low grade (G1–2), G3 and G4 as high grade (G3–4). In some tumour sites, no differentiation is made between G3 and G4, and therefore the category G3–4 is used. This is valid for carcinoma of the ovary, penis, prostate, kidney, renal pelvis, ureter, urinary bladder and urethra. Only three grades (G1–G3) are used for carcinoma of the uterine corpus, and malignant melanoma of the conjunctiva and uvea.

In carcinoma of the thyroid, pleural mesothelioma, malignant melanoma of the skin and of the eyelids, retinoblastoma, gestational trophoblastic tumours and malignant testicular tumours, grading is not applicable.

For undifferentiated carcinomas of the oesophagus, stomach, gallbladder, pancreas and colorectum, the category G4 is appropriate. By definition, an *adenocarcinoma* of these organs can be classified only as Gl, G2 or G3. When, in an adenocarcinoma of these organs, there are undifferentiated areas next to areas with glandular differentiation, the tumour is classified as a poorly differentiated adenocarcinoma (G3). The same applies for squamous cell carcinoma with undifferentiated areas.

In some sites the WHO classification lists no "undifferentiated carcinoma" as a specific tumour type, e.g., in lung and breast. In those cases, the category G4 is not applied [17].

In the absence of an assigned grade the following can be considered G4:

- Undifferentiated carcinoma (where provided)
- Small cell carcinoma
- Large cell carcinoma of lung
- Ewing sarcoma of bone and soft tissue
- Rhabdomyosarcoma of soft tissue

In grading, different methods may be appropriate for the various tumour entities (type and site). For example, in gastrointestinal adenocarcinomas the growing edge of a tumour should not be assessed because it may appear to be of high grade [31]; in contrast, grading that considers the histologically invasive edge is appropriate for predicting the prognosis of oral squamous cell carcinoma [5].

Grading is generally performed by a combined evaluation of various histological and cytological features, including similarity to tissue of origin, cell arrangement, cellularity, differentiation, cellular and nuclear pleomorphism, mitotic activity and necrosis. Grading is a semiquantitative, sometimes subjective procedure which requires considerable experience by the pathologist. To reduce individual variability and to increase reproducibility of grading, semiquantitative methods have been proposed. Various morphological parameters have been scored from 1 to 3 or 1 to 4, and the scores for each variable are added into a total malignancy score for each tumour. A high malignancy score suggests a poorly differentiated tumour. Such grading systems have been published, e.g., for breast carcinoma (Bloom and Richardson 1957 [4]; Schnürch et al. 1989 [51], Elston and Ellis 1991 [11], Pinder et al. 1998 [44]), soft tissue sarcomas (Costa et al. 1982 [8], Markhede et al. 1982 [36], Myhre-Jensen et al. 1983 [41], Coindre et al. 1986 [6]; Enzinger and Weiss 1988 [12]), prostate carcinoma (Gleason et al. 1977 [13]; Müller et al. 1980 [39]) and oral squamous cell carcinoma (Anneroth and Hansen 1984 [1], Anneroth et al. 1987 [2]; Bryne et al. 1989). The pathologist should indicate the grading system used in the report.

Note. Note. The various T, N and M categories as well as the categories of optional classifications like R, L, V, G should be written as common Arabic numerals, not as subscripts, e.g., T1 (not T_1) and N3 (not N_3). Stages are designated by Roman numerals.

References

[1] Anneroth G, Hansen LS. A methodologic study of histologic classification and grading of malignancy in oral squamous cell carcinoma. *Scand J Dent Res* 1984; **92**: 448–468

[2] Anneroth G, Batsakis J, Luna M. Review of the literature and a recommended system of malignancy grading in oral squamous cell carcinoma. *Scand J Dent Res* 1987; **95**: 229–249

[3] Becker K, Mueller J, Fink U, Matzen K, Sendler A, Dittler HJ, Helmberger H, Siewert JR, Höfler H. The interpretation of pathologic changes in the resection specimen following multimodal therapy for gastric adenocarcinomas. In *Progress in Gastric Cancer Research*, Siewert JR, Roder JD (eds) Monduzzi: Bologna, 1997; pp 1275–1280

[4] Bloom HJG, Richardson WW. Histologic grading and prognosis in breast cancer. *Br J Cancer* 1957; **11**: 359–377

[5] Bryne M, Koppang HS, Lilleng R, Stene T, Bang G, Dabelsteen E. New malignancy grading is a better prognostic indicator than Broder's grading in oral squamous cell carcinoma. *J Oral Pathol Med* 1989; **18**: 432–437

[6] Coindre JM, Trojani M, Contesso G et al.. Reproducibility of a histopathological grading system for adult soft tissue sarcoma. *Cancer* 1986; **58**: 306–309

[7] Compton C, Fenoglio-Preiser CM, Pettigrew N, Fielding LP. American Joint Committee on Cancer Prognostic Factors Consensus Conference: Colorectal Working group. *Cancer* 2000; **88**: 1739–1757

[8] Costa J, Wesley RA, Glatstein E, Rosenberg SA. The grading of soft tissue sarcomas: Results of a clinicopathological correlation in a series of 163 cases. *Cancer* 1982; **53**: 530–541

[9] Dudeck J, Wagner G, Grundmann E, Hermanek P Arbeitsgemeinschaft Deutscher Tumorzentren (ADT) Qualitätssicherung in der Onkologie. Basisdokumentation für Tumorkranke. Prinzipien und Verschlüsselungsanweisungen für Klinik und Praxis. 5. Aufl., Zuckschwerdt: München Bern Wien New York, 1999

[10] Dworak O, Keilholz L, Hoffmann A. Pathological features of rectal cancer after preoperative radiochemotherapy. *Int J Colorect Dis* 1997; **12**: 19–23

[11] Elston CW, Ellis LO. Pathological prognostic factors in breast cancer. I. The value of histological grade in breast cancer: experience from a large study with long-term follow-up. *Histopathology* 1991; **19**: 403–410

[12] Enzinger FM, Weiss SW. *Soft tissue tumors*, 3rd ed, Mosby, St. Louis, 1995

[13] Gleason DF, Veterans Administration Cooperative Urological Research Group (VACURG). Histologic grading and clinical staging of prostatic carcinoma. In *Urologic pathology: the prostate*. Tannenbaum M (ed) Lea and Fiebiger: Philadelphia, 1977

[14] Goldstein NS, Turner JR. Pericolonic tumors deposits in patients with T3N+M0 colon adenocarcinomas: a marker for reduced disease-free survival and intra-abdominal metastasis. *Cancer* 2000; **88**: 2228–2238

[15] Harrison JC, Dean PJ, El-Zeky F, Vander Zwaag R. From Dukes through Jass. Pathological prognostic indicators in rectal cancer. *Hum Pathol* 1994; **25**: 498–505

[16] Harrison JC, Dean PJ, El-Zeky F, Vander Zwaag R. Impact of the Crohn's like lymphoid reaction on staging of right-sided colon cancer. Results of a multivariate analysis. *Hum Pathol* 1995; **26**: 31–38

[17] Henson DE, Ries L, Freedman LS, Carriaga M. Relationship among outcome, stage of disease, and histologic grade for 22 616 cases of breast cancer. *Cancer* 1991; **68**: 2142–2149

[18] Hermanek P, Wittekind Ch. Residual Tumor (R) Classification and Prognosis. *Sem Surg Oncol* 1994; **10**: 12–20

[19] Hermanek P, Wittekind C. The pathologist and the Residual Tumor (R) classification. *Path Res Pract* 1994; **190**: 115–123

[20] Hermanek P, Wittekind Ch, Altendorf-Hofmann A. UICC Classification of pancreatic ductal adenocarcinoma. *Intern J Pancreatol* 1994; **16**: 230–232

[21] Hermanek P, Wittekind Ch. News of TNM and its use for classification of gastric cancer. *World J Surg* 1995; **19**: 491–495

[22] Hermanek P. pTNM and residual tumour classification: problems and prognostic factors. *World J Surg* 1995; **19**: 184–190

[23] Hermanek P. Staging systems. A review. In *Rectal cancer surgery. Optimisation–Standardisation–Documentation*. Soreide O, Norstein J (eds) Springer: Berlin Heidelberg New York Tokyo, 1997; pp 49–62

[24] Hermanek P, Bülzebruck H. Staging des Lungenkarzinoms. In *Thorax-tumoren. Diagnostik–Staging–gegenwärtiges Therapiekonzept.* Drings P, Vogt-Moykopf I (Hrsg) 2. Aufl. Springer: Berlin Heidelberg New York Tokyo, 1998 pp 97–117

[25] Hermanek P, Hutter RVP, Sobin LH, Wittekind Ch. Classification of isolated tumour cells and micrometastasis. *Cancer* 1999; **86**: 2668–2673

[26] Huvos AG. *Bone tumours. diagnosis, treatment and prognosis.* (2nd ed.) Saunders: Philadelphia London Toronto, 1991

[27] Jaehne J, Meyer HJ, Soudah B, Maschek HJ, Pichlmayr R. Peritoneal lavage in gastric carcinoma. *Dig Surg* 1989; **6**: 26–28

[28] Japanese Society for Esophageal Diseases. *Guidelines for the clinical and pathologic studies on carcinomas of the esophagus.* (8th ed.) Kanehara: Tokyo, 1990

[29] Japanese Research Society for Gastric Cancer (JRSGC) *Japanese classification of gastric carcinoma.* (1st English ed.). Nishi M, Omori Y, Miwa K (eds) Kanehara Shuppan, Tokyo, 1995

[30] Japanese Gastric Cancer Association (JGCA). Japanese classification of gastric carcinoma. 2nd English edition. *Gastric Cancer* 1998; **1**: 10–24

[31] Jass JR, Sobin LH. *Histological typing of intestinal tumours, 2nd ed, WHO International Histological Classification of Tumours.* Springer: Berlin Heidelberg New York, 1989

[32] Junker K, Krapp D, Müller KM. Kleinzelliges Bronchialkarzinom nach Chemotherapie–Morphologische Befunde. *Pathologe* 1995; **16**: 217–222

[33] Junker K, Thomas M, Schulmann K, Klinke V, Borse U, Müller KM. Regressionsgrading neoadjuvant behandelter nichtkleinzelliger Lungenkarzinome. *Pathologe* 1997; **18**: 131–140

[34] Klimpfinger M, Hauser H, Berger A, Hermanek P. Aktuelle klinische-pathologische Klassifikation von Karzinomen des Analkanals. *Acta Chir Aust* 1994; **26**: 345–351

[35] Mandard A-M, Dalibard F, Mandard JC, Marnay J, Henry-Amar M, Petiot J-F, Roussel A, et al.. Pathologic assessment of tumour regression after preoperative chemoradiotherapy of oesophgeal carcinoma. *Cancer* 1994; **73**: 2680–2696

[36] Markhede G, Angervall L, Stener B. A multivariate analysis of the prognosis after surgical treatment of malignant soft tissue tumours. *Cancer* 1982; **49**: 1721–1733

[37] Martin JK Jr, Goellner JR. Abdominal fluid cytology in patients with gastrointestinal malignant lesions. *Mayo Clin Proc* 1986; **61**: 467–471

[38] Maruyama K. Diagnosis of invisible peritoneal metastasis: cytologic examination by peritoneal lavage. In *Staging and Treatment of Gastric Cancer.* Cordine C, de Manzoni G (eds) Piccin Nuova Libraria: Padua, 1991; pp 180–181

[39] Müller HA, Altemähr E, Böcking A, Dhom G, Faul P, Göttinger H, Helpap B, Hohbach C, Kastendieck H, Leistenschneider G. Über Klassifikation und Grading des Prostatacarcinomas. *Verh Dtsch Ges Path* 1980; **64**: 609–611

[40] Müller KM, Wiethege Th, Junker K. Pathologie kleinzelliger Lungentumoren. *Onkologe* 1998; **4**: 996–1001

[41] Myhre-Jensen O, Kaae S, Hjollund Madsen E, Sneppen O. Histopathological grading in soft tissue tumours: Relation to survival in 261 surgically treated patients. *Acta Path Microbiol Immunol Scand (Sect A)* 1983; **91**: 145–150

[42] Nakajima T, Harashima S, Hirata M, Kajitani T. Prognostic and therapeutic values of peritoneal cytology in gastric cancer. *Acta Cytol* 1978; **22**: 225–229

[43] Pantel K, Coste RJ, Fodstad O. Detection and clinical importance of micrometastatic disease. *J Natl Cancer Inst* 1999; **91**: 1113–1124

[44] Pinder SE, Murray S, Ellis IO, Trihia H, Elston CW, Gelber RD, Goldhirsch A, Lindtner J, Cortés-Funes H, Simoncii E, Byrne MJ, Golouh R, Rudenstam CM, Castiglione-Gertsch M. Gusterson BA. The importance of histologic grade of invasive breast carcinoma and response to chemotherapy. *Cancer* 1998; **83**: 1529–1533

[45] Quirke P, Dixon MF. The prediction of the local recurrence in rectal adenocarcinoma by histopathological examination. *Int J Colorectal Dis* 1988; **3**: 127–131

[46] Quirke P. The pathologist, the surgeon and colorectal cancer–get it right because it matters. *Prog Pathol* 1998; **4**: 201–213

[47] Salzer-Kuntschik M, Delling G, Beron G, Sigmund R. Morphological grades of regression in osteosarcoma after polychemotherapy–Study Case 80. *J Cancer Res Clin Pract* 1993; **106**, Suppl: 21–24

[48] Scheele J, Stangl R, Altendorf-Hofmann A, Gall FP. Indicators of prognosis after hepatic resection for colorectal secondaries. *Surgery* 1990; **110**: 13–29

[49] Schlimok G, Funke I, Pantel K, et al.. Micrometastatic tumour cells in bone marrow of patients with gastric cancer: methodological aspects of detection and clinical significance. *Eur J Cancer* 1991; **27**: 1461–1465

[50] Schmidt RA, Conrad EU, Collins C, Rabinovitch P, Finney A. Measurement and prediction of short-term response of soft tissue sarcomas to chemotherapy. *Cancer* 1993; **72**: 2593–2601

[51] Schnürch HG, Lange C, Bender HG. Vier histopathologische Differenzierungsgrade beim Mammakarzinom? *Pathologe* 1989; **10**: 39–42

[52] SEER Program: *Code manual, Third edition.* NIH Publication No 98-2313. National Cancer Institute: Bethesda, 1998.

[53] Sinn HP, Schmid H, Junkermann H, Houber J, Leppien G, Kaufmann M, Bastert G et al.. Histologische Regression des Mammakarzinoms nach

primärer (neoadjuvanter) Chemotherapie. *Geburtsh Frauenheilk* 1994; **34**: 332–338

[54] Veronesi U, Farante G, Galimberti V, Greco M, Luini A, Sacchini V, Andreola S, Leoni F, Menard S, Ronco M, Colnaghi MI. Evaluation of resection margins after breast conservative surgery with monoclonal antibodies. *Eur J Surg Oncol* 1991; **17**: 338–341

[55] Warshaw AL. Implications of peritoneal cytology for staging of early pancreatic cancer. *Am J Surg* 1991; **161**: 26–30

[56] Zeng Z, Cohen AM, Haydu S, Sternberg SS, Sigurdson ER, Enker W. Serosal cytologic study to determine free mesothelial penetration by intraperitoneal colon cancer. *Cancer* 1992; **70**: 737–740

Explanatory Notes–Specific Anatomical Sites

Head and Neck Tumours

General

Anatomy

A uniform topographic terminology should be used for classification, and the "sites, subsites, adjacent sites and adjacent structures" should be used as defined in the text.

Tumours involving two anatomical sites are classified according to the site in which the greater part of the tumour is located. In invasive tumours with an associated carcinoma in situ, only the invasive component is considered for classification.

Example. Carcinoma with two-thirds in the hypopharynx and one-third in the supraglottis is classified as hypopharynx carcinoma.

Extension to Adjacent Sites

In tumours extending to an adjacent site, differentiation between superficial extension and deep extension is necessary. In superficial extension, the involvement is limited to the mucosa; in deep extension, muscles, bones or other deep structures are invaded.

Superficial extension to adjacent sites is not considered invasion of adjacent structures (T4).

Example. A tumour extending from the oropharynx to nasopharynx or hypopharynx or to oral cavity and limited to the mucosa (without invasion of muscles, bones or other deep structures) is classified only according to size. The involvement of nasopharynx or hypopharynx or oral cavity is not considered invasion of adjacent structures as long as the tumour is limited to the mucosa.

Deep extension to an adjacent site can be the result of vertical invasion of adjacent structures (see above) or the result of horizontal spread *not* limited to the mucosa but also involving muscles or bones. Such extension is classified as invasion of adjacent structures (T4).

23

Example. Base of tongue carcinoma invading the preepiglottic space is classified as T4.

Adjacent Structures

Adjacent structures refer to organs and tissues that can be deeply invaded by a tumour, e.g., extension of a glottis carcinoma through thyroid cartilage into soft tissues of the neck or extension of a carcinoma of the maxillary sinus into the orbit.

Regional Lymph Nodes

According to the *TNM Atlas* [31] the cervical lymph nodes include the following groups (Figs. 2 and 3. See also Fig. 1, p. 22 of the AJCC manual [1]):
The first 8 groups are commonly referred to by levels:

1. Submental nodes (Level IA)
2. Submandibular nodes (syn. submaxillary nodes) (Level IB)
3. Cranial jugular (deep cervical) nodes (Level II)
4. Medial jugular (deep cervical) nodes (Level III)
5. Caudal jugular (deep cervical) nodes (Level IV)
6. Dorsal cervical (superficial cervical) nodes along the spinal accessory nerve (Level V)
7. Supraclavicular nodes (Level IV and, uncommonly, Level V)
8. Prelaryngeal and paratracheal (syn. anterior cervical) nodes (Level VI)
9. Retropharyngeal nodes
10. Parotid nodes
11. Buccal nodes (syn. facial nodes)
12. Retroauricular (syn. mastoid, posterior auricular) and occipital nodes

   In 1991, a standardized neck dissection terminology was published by a Committee for Head and Neck Surgery and Oncology of the American Academy for Otolaryngology–Head and Neck Surgery [24]. In October 1992, at an international symposium in Göttingen, Germany, this terminology was accepted by representatives of various European cancer centers (Villejuif, Milan, Amsterdam). We support the use of this terminology [24]. The lymph node groups 1–8 are defined as follows:

1. Submental group (Level IA):
   Lymph nodes within the triangular boundary of the anterior belly of the digastric muscle and the hyoid bone.
2. Submandibular group (Level IB):
   Lymph nodes within the boundaries of the anterior and posterior bellies of the digastric muscle and the body of the mandible.
3. Upper jugular group (Level II):
   Lymph nodes located around the upper third of the internal jugular vein and adjacent spinal accessory nerve, extending from the hyoid bone (clinical

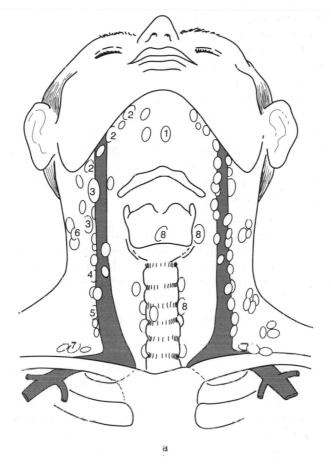

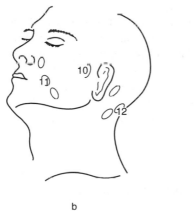

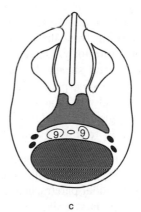

Figure 2. Cervical lymph node groups [31]

landmark) to the skull base. The posterior boundary is the posterior border of the sternocleidomastoid muscle, and the anterior boundary is the lateral border of the sternohyoid muscle. This group includes the jugulodigastric node, which is the most cranial jugular node.

4. Middle jugular group (Level III):
   Lymph nodes located around the middle third of the internal jugular vein, extending from the carotid bifurcation superiorly to the omohyoid muscle (surgical landmark) or cricothyroid notch (clinical landmark) inferiorly. The posterior boundary is the posterior border of the sternocleidomastoid muscle, and the anterior boundary is the lateral border of the sternohyoid muscle. This group includes the juguloomohyoid node located between omohyoid muscle and internal jugular vein.

5. Lower jugular group (Level IV):
   Lymph nodes located around the lower third of the internal jugular vein, extending from the omohyoid muscle superiorly to the clavicle inferiorly. The posterior boundary is the posterior border of the sternocleidomastoid muscle, and the anterior boundary is the lateral border of the sternohyoid muscle.

6. Dorsal cervical nodes along the spinal accessory nerve (Level V) and

7. Supraclavicular nodes (mostly Level IV):
   The two groups are combined and called the "posterior triangle group": This comprises predominantly the lymph nodes located along the lower half of the spinal accessory nerve and the transverse cervical artery. The supraclavicular nodes are also included. The posterior boundary is the anterior border of the trapezius muscle, the anterior boundary is the posterior border of the sternocleidomastoid muscle, and the inferior border is the clavicle. Most are in Level IV; some may occupy the most caudal component of Level V.

8. Anterior compartment group (Level VI):
   Lymph nodes surrounding the midline visceral structures of the neck, extending from the level of the hyoid bone superiorly to the suprasternal notch inferiorly. On each side, the lateral boundary is the medial border of the carotid sheath. Located within this compartment are the perithyroidal lymph nodes, paratracheal lymph nodes, lymph nodes along the recurrent laryngeal nerves and precricoid lymph nodes.
   Node group 8 (prelaryngeal and paratracheal nodes) may be further subdivided as follows (Figure 3):

   - 8a: cranial paratracheal (suprathyroidal)
   - 8b: thyroidal (perithyroidal)
   - 8c: caudal paratracheal (infrathyroidal, lateral tracheal)
   - 8d: prelaryngeal
   - 8e: pretracheal near the thyroid isthmus (delphian)

Level (Robbins et al. [24])	Lymph node group number	Lymph node terminology TNM Atlas [31]	Robbins et al. [24]
I	1	Submental nodes	Submental group
	2	Submandibular nodes	Submandibular group
II	3	Cranial jugular nodes	Upper jugular group
III	4	Medial jugular nodes	Middle jugular group
IV	5	Caudal jugular nodes	Lower jugular group
V	6	Dorsal cervical nodes along the accessory nerve	Posterior triangle group
IV, V	7	Supraclavicular nodes	
VI	8	Prelaryngeal and paratracheal nodes	Anterior compartment group

9. Retropharyngeal nodes
10. *The parotid nodes* may be subdivided into superficial (in front of tragus on top of parotid fascia) and deep parotid nodes. The latter are located underneath the parotid fascia and include intraglandular nodes directly in parotid gland. The preauricular and infra-auricular (infra- or subparotid) nodes are assigned to the parotid nodes.
11. *The buccal (facial) nodes* include the buccinator nodes located deep on buccinator muscle, the nasolabial nodes located underneath nasolabial groove, the molar nodes located in the surface of cheek and the mandibular nodes located outside the lower jaw.

For thyroid surgery, a distinction between a central and a lateral compartment is of interest for treatment planning [5]. The central compartment includes groups 1, 2 and 8, the lateral compartment groups 3–7.

The regional lymph nodes for thyroid include the *upper mediastinal lymph nodes*, which may be subdivided into tracheo-oesophageal (posterior mediastinal) and upper anterior mediastinal nodes. Cervical and mediastinal lymph nodes are not divided by a fascia; the left brachiocephalic vein is considered to be the boundary [5].

N Classification

Size of Lymph Nodes: In advanced lymphatic spread, one often finds perinodal tumour and the confluence of several lymph node metastases into one large tumour conglomerate. In the definition of the N classification, the perinodal component should be included in the size for isolated lymph node metastases; for conglomerates, the overall size of the conglomerate should be considered and not only the size of the individual lymph nodes.

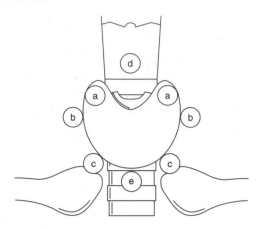

Figure 3. Subdivision of prelaryngeal and paratracheal (anterior cervical) lymph nodes (group 8).

Lip and Oral Cavity

Summary Lip, Oral Cavity

T1	≤2 cm
T2	>2–4 cm
T3	>4 cm
T4	Adjacent structures

Lip

Tumours that affect the vermilion surface as well as the skin are assigned to the lip when 50% or more of the tumour is within the vermilion surface.

The vermilion surface is demarcated from the mucosal surface by the line of contact of the opposing lips.

Skin of face is not classified as an adjacent structure.

Invasion up to cortical bone or erosion of the bone is not classified T4. There must be invasion through the cortical bone into the spongiosa.

Oral Cavity

1. T4 definitions:
   a) The deep (extrinsic) muscle of the tongue includes musculi hyo-, stylo-, genio- and palatoglossus. Invasion indicates T4. Generally, deep muscle invasion is associated with restriction of mobility of the tongue when examined clinically.
   b) The intrinsic muscle of the tongue includes musculi longitudinalis superior and inferior, transversus linguae and verticalis linguae. Invasion of the intrinsic muscle alone or the submandibular gland is not classified T4.

c) Invasion up to cortical bone or erosion of the bone is not classified T4. There must be invasion through the cortical bone into the spongiosa.

d) Invasion of the sublingual gland by a carcinoma of the floor of mouth does not qualify for T4 and is not considered in the T classification.

2. A tumour extending from the oral cavity to the oropharynx and limited to the mucosa (without invasion of muscles, bones or other deep structures) is classified only according to size. The involvement of oropharynx is not considered invasion of adjacent structures as long as the tumour is limited to the mucosa.

Pharynx

Oropharynx

Summary Oropharynx

T1	≤ 2 cm
T2	$>2-4$ cm
T3	>4 cm
T4	Adjacent structures

A tumour extending from the oropharynx to the nasopharynx or to the hypopharynx or to the oral cavity or larynx and limited to the mucosa (without invasion of muscles, bones or other deep structures) is classified only according to size up to T3. The involvement of nasopharynx or hypopharynx or oral cavity or larynx is not considered invasion of adjacent structures provided that the tumour is limited to the mucosa.

A tumour invading soft tissue of neck and paravertebral fascia/muscles is classified as T4.

Definition of invasion of the larynx: Invasion of outer framework (thyroid cartilage, cricoid cartilage, preepiglottic space) or internal structures such as arytenoid and epiglottic cartilages.

Nasopharynx

Summary Nasopharynx

T1		Nasopharynx
T2		Soft tissue of oropharynx and/or nasal fossa
	T2a	Without parapharyngeal extension
	T2b	With parapharyngeal extension
T3		Invades bony structures and/or paranasal sinuses
T4		Intracranial extension, involvement of cranial nerves, infratemporal fossa, hypopharynx, orbit

Tumours not involving the oropharynx and/or nasal fossa but with parapharyngeal extension are classified T2b.

The term "postnasal space" corresponds to nasopharynx (C11). Invasion of vertebral bodies is classified T3.

The terms masticator space and infratemporal fossa are considered synonymous here.

Hypopharynx

Summary Hypopharynx

T1	≤2 cm and limited to one subsite
T2	>2 to 4 cm or more than one subsite
T3	>4 cm or with larynx fixation
T4	Invades adjacent structures

1. The term "laryngopharynx" corresponds to hypopharynx (C13.9).
2. For classification, the hypopharyngeal surface of the aryepiglottic fold (C13.1) belongs to the hypopharynx, whereas the laryngeal aspect of the aryepiglottic fold (C32.1) is part of the supraglottis.
3. Fixation of hemilarynx is diagnosed endoscopically by immobility of the arytenoid or vocal cord.
4. The uncommon tumours limited to one subsite but with vocal cord fixation should be classified as T3.
5. Involvement of the arytenoid cartilage is classified as T3, not T4.
6. Invasion of adjacent structures (T4) includes (see also p. 24)
   - Invasion of the thyroid cartilage or cricoid cartilage (involvement of perichondrium only is not invasion of the cartilage)
   - Invasion of the soft tissues of the neck
   - Invasion of vertebral bodies
7. A tumour extending from the hypopharynx to oesophagus and limited to the mucosa (without invasion of muscles, bones or other deeper structures) is classified only according to size up to T3.
8. A tumour of the sinus piriformis (C12.9) with invasion of the thyroid cartilage should not be classified as T4 but rather as T3.

Larynx

Summary Larynx

Summary Supraglottis

T1	One subsite, normal mobility
T2	Involving mucosa of more than one adjacent subsite of supraglottis or glottis or adjacent region outside the supraglottis, without fixation

| T3 | Limited to the larynx with vocal cord fixation or invades postcricoid area, pre-epiglottic tissues, base of tongue |
| T4 | Extends beyond the larynx |

Summary Glottis

T1	Limited to vocal cord(s), normal mobility
T2	Supraglottis, subglottis, impaired cord mobility
T3	Cord fixation
T4	Extends beyond larynx

Summary Subglottis

T1	Limited to the subglottis
T2	Extends to vocal cord(s) with normal/ impaired mobility
T3	Cord fixation
T4	Extends beyond larynx

Anatomical Definitions

Superior and Inferior Boundaries of the Glottis

According to the *AJCC Cancer Staging Manual* [1], the inferior boundary of the supraglottis is the horizontal plane passing through the lateral margin of the ventricle at its junction with the superior surface of the vocal cord. Kleinsasser [19, 20] emphasized embryological and functional reasons for the following definition of the boundary between supraglottis and glottis:

A plane running horizontally through the opening of the ventricle, posteriorly over the vocal process of the arytenoid cartilage and then rising between the cuneiform and the corniculate cartilage to end over the upper edge of the posterior commissure.

According to the *AJCC Cancer Staging Manual* [1], the lower boundary of the glottis is the horizontal plane 1 cm below the lateral margin of the ventricle.

According to Alberti u. Boyce [2] the following definition is recommended: The inferior boundary of the glottis is a horizontal plane 1 cm inferior to the level of the upper surface of the vocal cords, which divides supraglottis and glottis (Fig. 54 *TNM Atlas* 1997 [31]).

Pathological Criteria of Impaired Vocal Cord Mobility or Vocal Cord Fixation

Impaired Mobility or Fixation

For pathological classification concerning impaired mobility or fixation of vocal cords the information from the clinical T is used for the pathologic T. This is in accordance with TNM rule No. 2, pathological classification "is based on the evidence acquired before treatment, supplemented or modified by the additional evidence acquired from surgery and from pathological examination".

Associated Carcinoma In Situ

1. For invasive carcinoma, the classification according to horizontal spread is based only on the invasive component.
2. To indicate the presence of associated carcinoma in situ (adjacent or separate) the suffix "(is)" may be added to the respective T category of the invasive carcinoma, e.g., T2(is). The presence of an associated carcinoma in situ influences treatment of the invasive carcinoma and needs identification and separate analysis of such cases.

Paranasal Sinuses

Summary Maxillary Sinus

T1	Antral mucosa
T2	Bone destruction
T3	Posterior wall maxillary sinus, subcutaneous tissues, skin of cheek, floor/medial wall of orbit, infratemporal fossa, pterygoid plates, ethmoid sinus(es)
T4	Orbital contents, cribriform plate, base of skull, nasopharynx, sphenoid, frontal sinus

Summary Ethmoid Sinus

T1	Ethmoid (with or without bone erosion)
T2	Nasal cavity
T3	Anterior orbit, maxillary sinus
T4	Intracranial cavity, orbital apex, sphenoid, frontal sinus, skin of nose

Erosion of bone indicates that the tumour invades the cortex only; *invasion* of bone indicates that the spongiosa is involved.

Salivary Glands

Summary Salivary Glands

T1	≤2 cm, without extraparenchymal extension
T2	>2 to 4 cm, without extraparenchymal extension
T3	Extraparenchymal extension, and/or >4 to 6 cm
T4	Base of skull, seventh nerve, and/or >6 cm

Tumours arising in minor salivary glands localized to the mucous membrane of the upper aerodigestive tract are classified according to the rules for tumours of the oral cavity or pharynx.

Designation by histological type should be done to permit separation of squamous mucosal tumours from salivary gland tumours.

Digestive System Tumours

Rules for Classification

The classification applies to all types of carcinoma including small cell carcinoma. It does not apply to carcinoids.

Oesophagus

Summary Oesophagus

T1	Lamina propria, submucosa
T2	Muscularis propria
T3	Adventitia
T4	Adjacent structures
N1	Regional
M1	Distant metastasis
	Tumour of lower thoracic oesophagus
M1a	Coeliac nodes
M1b	Other distant metastasis
	Tumour of upper thoracic oesophagus
M1a	Cervical nodes
M1b	Other distant metastasis
	Tumour of mid-thoracic oesophagus
M1b	Distant metastasis including nonregional nodes

There is a proposal to divide carcinomas of the oesophago-gastric junction region into three entities [27, 28]:

- adenocarcinoma of the distal oesophagus (adenocarcinoma of the esophagogastric junction = AEG I, Barrett)
- "real" carcinoma of the cardia (AEG II)
- subcardial carcinoma of the stomach, infiltrating the distal oesophagus (AEG III)

Nevertheless, there exists no separate TNM classification for tumours of the cardia. For discussion of tumours of the cardia, see below, stomach anatomy.

For tumours of the lower and upper oesophagus, the categories M1a and M1b are provided:

Lower thoracic oesophagus:

M1a   Metastasis in coeliac lymph nodes
M1b   Other distant metastasis

Upper thoracic oesophagus:

M1a   Metastasis in cervical lymph nodes
M1b   Other distant metastasis

In contrast, for tumours of mid-thoracic oesophagus, any distant metastasis is classified as M1b. For tumours of cervical oesophagus only the category M1 (without subdivision) is used.

Stomach

Anatomy

Gastric tumours located in the cardiac area may involve the distal oesophagus and primary oesophageal tumours may involve the cardiac area of the stomach. For differentiation between oesophageal and gastric carcinomas the following may be considered:

- If more than 50% of the tumour involves the oesophagus, the tumour is classified as oesophageal; if less than 50%, as gastric
- If the tumour is equally located above and below the oesophagogastric junction or is designated as being at the junction, squamous cell, small cell and undifferentiated carcinomas are classified as oesophageal, adenocarcinoma and signet ring cell carcinoma as gastric
- In the presence of Barrett oesophagus, an adenocarcinoma in both cardia and lower oesophagus is most likely to be oesophageal. In the absence of Barrett oesophagus such an adenocarcinoma is most likely to be gastric.

Regional Lymph Nodes

The regional lymph nodes are:
- The perigastric nodes along the lesser curvature

    1   Right cardiac
    3   Lesser curvature
    5   Suprapyloric

- The perigastric nodes along the greater curvature

    2   Left cardiac
    4a   Greater curvature left
    4b   Greater curvature right
    6   Infrapyloric

- The nodes located along the main trunks of the following arteries

7	Left gastric
8	Common hepatic
9	Coeliac
10	Splenic/at the splenic hilum
11	Splenic/along trunk
12	Nodes in the hepatoduodenal ligament

Note. The numerical order corresponds to the proposals of the Japanese Research Society for Gastric Cancer [17].

Nomenclature of the 2nd ed. Japanese Classification [18]

Perigastric Lymph Nodes

No. 1   Right paracardial
No. 2   Left paracardial
No. 3   Along the lesser curvature
No. 4   Along the greater curvature
(According to the TNM Atlas this station may be subdivided into 4a left and 4b right)
No. 5   Suprapyloric
No. 6   Infrapyloric

Lymph Nodes of the Gastric Bed

No. 7   Along the left gastric artery
No. 8   Along the common hepatic artery
No. 9   Around the celiac artery
No. 10   At the splenic hilum
No. 11   Along the splenic artery
No. 12   In the hepatoduodenal ligament

Note. The numerical order corresponds to the proposals of the Japanese Gastric Cancer Association [18].

Stations 7, 8, 9 and 11 ("along the. . .", around the . . .") include only lymph nodes along the main trunk of the mentioned arteries. Lymph nodes along the ramifications of the left gastric artery are classified as perigastric nodes.

In case of gastric stump carcinoma (after previous distal gastrectomy and localized at the anastomosis), lymph nodes in the mesentery of the intestinal loop used for anastomosis are classified as gastric regional nodes.

In case of invasion of the oesophagus the infradiaphragmatic lymph nodes (no. 19) and the lymph nodes of the oesophageal hiatus (no. 20) are considered as additional regional lymph nodes [18].

T Classification

Summary Stomach

T1	Lamina propria, submucosa
T2	Muscularis propria
T3	Penetrates serosa
T4	Adjacent structures

Invasion of the transverse mesocolon is considered analogous to invasion of the gastrocolic ligament and is therefore classified T2 if the covering visceral peritoneum is not perforated (see *TNM Classification* 1997 [30], Note 1, p. 60). The same applies to direct invasion of the greater omentum. Tumour nodules in the greater omentum that are separate from the primary tumour are classified as distant (peritoneal) metastasis (M1 PER).

Small Intestine

Summary Small Intestine

T1	Lamina propria, submucosa
T2	Muscularis propria
T3	Subserosa, nonperitonealized perimuscular tissues (mesentery, retroperitoneum) ≤ 2 cm
T4	Visceral peritoneum, other organs/structures (including mesentery, retroperitoneum >2 cm)

The very uncommon carcinoma in a Meckel diverticulum may be classified according to the classification for small intestine carcinoma, although supporting data are not available.

Intramural extension of an ileal carcinoma directly into the caecum (not by way of the serosa) does not affect the T classification, in particular does not qualify for T4.

Colon and Rectum

Anatomical Sites and Subsites

1. A tumour located at the border between two subsites is registered as a tumour of the subsite that is more involved.

   Example. Carcinoma with a longitudinal diameter of 6 cm, 2 cm in the caecum, 4 cm in the ascending colon, is classified as a carcinoma of the ascending colon (C18.2).

   If two subsites are involved to the same extent, the lesion is classified as an overlapping lesion.

Example. If the carcinoma involves 2 cm of the caecum and 2 cm of the ascending colon, the code C18.8 (overlapping lesion of the colon) is used.

2. The rectum is defined as the distal large intestine commencing opposite the sacral promontory and ending at the upper border of the anal canal. When measured from below with a rigid sigmoidoscope, it extends 16 cm from the anal verge. A tumour is classified as rectal if its lower margin lies 16 cm or less from the anal verge [6, 29]. A tumour is considered rectal if any part is located at least partly within the supply of the superior rectal artery. Tumours are classified as rectosigmoid when differentiation between rectum and sigmoid according to the above rules is not possible.

Local Recurrence

A local recurrence after previous colon resection should be classified with the prefix "r"(for recurrence); the recurrent tumour is topographically assigned to the proximal segment of the anastomosis.

Regional Lymph Nodes

For each anatomical subsite the nodes along the following vessels (trunks and branches) are regional nodes:

Appendix	Ileocolic
Caecum	Ileocolic and right colic
Ascending colon	Ileocolic, right colic and middle colic
Hepatic flexure	Middle colic and right colic
Transverse colon	Right colic, middle colic, left colic and inferior mesenteric
Splenic flexure	Middle colic, left colic and inferior mesenteric
Descending colon	Left colic and inferior mesenteric
Sigmoid colon	Sigmoid, left colic, superior rectal (haemorrhoidal)
and rectosigmoid	and inferior mesenteric
Rectum	Superior rectal (haemorrhoidal), inferior mesenteric and internal iliac

Metastasis in nodes other than those listed above is classified as distant metastasis, e.g., metastasis in a node along the trunk of the middle colic artery and/or its ramification in a case of rectal carcinoma is M1. However, in case of direct (intramural) extension of the primary tumour to an adjacent subsite, the lymph nodes of the latter subsite are also considered regional lymph nodes.

Perirectal nodes include the mesorectal (paraproctal), lateral sacral, presacral, sacral promotory (Gerota), middle rectal (haemorrhoidal) and inferior rectal (haemorrhoidal) nodes. Metastasis in the external iliac or common iliac nodes is classified as distant metastasis (M1).

The pericolic nodes correspond to "epicolic," "paracolic" and "intermediate" nodes according to the division of Jamieson and Dobson [16] ("epicolic," and the colon itself; "paracolic" along the marginal artery and between it and the colon; "intermediate" nodes on the branches of the major colic vessels as well as nodes along the trunks of these vessels). The "principal glands" of Jamieson and

Dobson include the nodes on the inferior mesenteric artery and on the superior mesenteric artery, the latter to be classified as nonregional.

In case of direct invasion of the small intestine, lymph nodes in the mesentery of the invaded intestinal loop are classified as regional lymph nodes.

T/pT Classification

Summary Colon and Rectum

T1	Submucosa
T2	Muscularis propria
T3	Subserosa, nonperitonealized pericolic/perirectal tissues
T4	Other organs or structures/visceral peritoneum

Tumours of the appendix are classified using the TNM scheme for colon and rectum, but are analyzed separately.

According to a proposal of the AJCC (Yarbro et al., AJCC on Cancer Prognostic Factors Consensus Conference. Cancer 1999; 86: 2436–2446) the classification should not be applied to tumours of the appendix.

1. For colon and rectum only, Tis/pTis (carcinoma in situ) includes cases with invasion of the lamina propria (including the muscularis mucosae but not of the submucosa), i.e., intramucosal, as well as intraepithelial carcinoma.
2. T3/pT3: The perirectal tissue includes the mesorectum (paraproctium).
3. Tumour extension into the peritoneal cavity is classified as T4. Perforation of the visceral peritoneum at the microscopic level requires identification of tumour directly extending to and growing on the peritoneal surface and/or positive cytology on specimens obtained by scraping the serosa overlying the primary tumour [32].
4. *Intramural* direct extension from one subsite (segment) of the colon to an adjacent one is not considered in the T classification. The same applies to *intramural* direct extension from the rectum to the sigmoid colon and vice versa and from the rectum to the anal canal.
5. *Intramural* extension of a caecal carcinoma directly into the ileum (not by way of serosa) does not affect the T classification, in particular does not qualify for T4. In contrast, direct extension via serosa or via mesocolon is classified T4, e.g., extension of a sigmoid colon carcinoma to caecum.
6. Tumour cells in veins or lymphatics do not affect the pT classification. The L and V classifications can be used to record such spread (see also p. 39, N/pN classification).

    Example. Carcinoma with continuous local spread into the submucosa, tumour cells in a small vein within the muscularis propria - pT1, V1 (muscularis propria).

7. Invasion of the external sphincter should be classified as pT3.
8. Invasion of levator muscle(s) is classified as T4.

9. A tumour nodule in the soft tissues beneath a perineal operation skin scar after abdominoperineal resection for rectal carcinoma after a disease-free interval is classified as rT(+) not M1.

N/pN Classification

A tumour nodule greater than 3 mm in the perirectal or pericolic adipose tissue of a primary carcinoma without histological evidence of residual lymph node in the nodule is classified in the pN category as a regional lymph node metastasis if the nodule has the form and smooth contour of a lymph node. If the nodule has an irregular contour, it should be classified in the T or pT category and also coded as V1 (microscopic venous invasion) or V2, if it was grossly evident, because there is a strong likelihood that it arises from venous invasion. [12, 13, 14].

Involvement of the apical node(s) does not influence the N/pN classification.

M Classification

Tumour nodule(s) in an abdominal scar after removal of an intraabdominal tumour (with a disease-free interval) should be classified as M1, e.g., rT0 N0 M1 SKI.

Anal Canal

Rules for Classification

The classification applies to all types of carcinoma including those arising within an anorectal fistula as well as squamous cell (cloacogenic) carcinoma.

T Classification
Summary Anal Canal

T1	≤2 cm
T2	>2 to 5 cm
T3	>5 cm
T4	Adjacent organs

Involvement of the sphincter muscle(s) alone is not classified as T4.

Direct invasion of rectal wall or perirectal skin or subcutaneous perianal tissue is not considered T4. The tumour is classified by size.

Liver

Rules for Classification

The classification applies to intrahepatic cholangiocarcinoma (peripheral bile duct carcinoma) as well as hepatocellular carcinoma and combined hepatocellular and cholangiocarcinoma.

Regional Lymph Nodes

The regional lymph nodes are the hilar, hepatic (along the proper hepatic artery) and periportal (along the portal vein) nodes. In addition, the nodes along the abdominal inferior vena cava above the renal veins, except the inferior phrenic nodes are considered regional. Involvement of the inferior phrenic nodes (lymph nodes in the oesophageal hiatus of the diaphragm) should be considered M1.This expands the definition of regional nodes described in the original printing of the 5th edition of TNM and corresponds to the definition in the AJCC Cancer Staging Manual. It is supported by a study of Nozaki et al. [22].

T/pT Classification

Summary Liver

T1	Solitary, ≤2 cm, without vascular invasion
T2	Solitary, ≤2 cm, with vascular invasion
	Multiple, one lobe, ≤2 cm, without vascular invasion
	Solitary, >2 cm, without vascular invasion
T3	Solitary, >2 cm, with vascular invasion
	Multiple, one lobe, ≤2 cm, with vascular invasion
	Multiple, one lobe, >2 cm, with or without vascular invasion
T4	Multiple, more than one lobe
	Invasion of major branch of portal or hepatic veins
	Invasion of adjacent organs other than gallbladder
	Perforation of visceral peritoneum

1. "Multiplicity" includes multiple nodules representing multiple, independent primary tumours and intrahepatic metastasis from a single primary hepatic carcinoma
2. "Vascular invasion" is diagnosed clinically by imaging procedures. In the pathological assessment it includes gross and/or histological involvement of vessels including invasion of adventitia of major branches of vessels,
3. T4: "major branches of the portal or hepatic veins" are the right and left branches of the portal vein and the corresponding hepatic veins (not segmental or subsegmental branches). Involvement of the right, left and (not always existent) intermediate branches of the hepatic artery is also classified T4.

Gallbladder

Summary Gallbladder

T1		Lamina propria and muscle
	T1a	Lamina propria
	T1b	Muscle
T2		Perimuscular connective tissue

T3	Serosa and/or one organ, liver ≤ 2 cm
T4	Two or more organs, liver >2 cm

Carcinoma of the cystic duct is classified as a tumour of the extrahepatic bile ducts.

Extrahepatic Bile Ducts

Summary Extrahepatic Bile Ducts

T1		Ductal wall
	T1a	Subepithelial connective tissue
	T1b	Fibromuscular layer
T2		Perifibromuscular connective tissue
T3		Adjacent structures

Carcinoma of the cystic duct and carcinoma in a choledochal cyst are classified as extrahepatic bile duct tumours.

This classification does not apply to carcinomas of the ampulla of Vater.

Anatomical Subsites

The extrahepatic bile ducts include:
- Left and right hepatic ducts (tumours arising here are often referred to as hilar carcinomas of the liver, also named Klatskin tumours)
- Common hepatic duct
- Cystic duct
- Common bile duct (choledochus)

Direct invasion of the portal vein or the hepatic artery is classified T3.

Ampulla of Vater

The ampulla opens into the duodenum through a small mucosal elevation, the duodenal papilla or papilla of Vater. Tumours of the ampulla of Vater include tumours arising in the ampulla, tumours arising on the papilla and tumours arising at the junction of the mucosa of the ampulla with that of the papilla.

Pancreas (exocrine tumours only)

This classification is not applicable to tumours in aberrant pancreatic tissue.

Summary Pancreas

T1	Limited to the pancreas ≤ 2 cm
T2	Limited to the pancreas >2 cm

| T3 | Duodenum bile duct, peripancreatic tissues |
| T4 | Stomach, spleen, colon, large vessels |

T Classification

T3 Peripancreatic tissues include the surrounding retroperitoneal fat (retroperitoneal soft tissue or retroperitoneal space), including the mesentery (mesenteric fat), mesocolon, greater and lesser omentum and peritoneum.
Direct invasion to bile ducts and duodenum includes involvement of the ampulla of Vater.

T4 Adjacent large vessels are the portal vein, the coeliac artery and the superior mesenteric and common hepatic arteries and veins.

Regional Lymph Nodes

There are some differences in the designation of regional lymph nodes between the UICC and AJCC classifications, see appendix , p. 59ff.

Lung

Rules for Classification

The classification applies to all types of carcinoma including small cell carcinoma. It does not apply to carcinoids.

T Classification
Summary Lung

T1	≤3 cm
T2	>3 cm, main bronchus ≥2 cm from carina, invades visceral pleura, partial atelectasis
T3	Chest wall, diaphragm, pericardium, mediastinal pleura Main bronchus <2 cm from carina, total atelectasis
T4	Mediastinum, heart, great vessels, carina, trachea, oesophagus, vertebra; separate nodules in same lobe, malignant effusion

1. Tumour with local invasion of another lobe without tumour on the pleural surface should be classified as T2.
2. Invasion of phrenic nerve is classified as T3.
3. Vocal cord paralysis (resulting from invasion of the recurrent branch of the vagus nerve), superior vena caval obstruction or compression of the trachea or oesophagus is classified as T4.
4. T4: the "great vessels" are
   - Aorta
   - Superior vena cava
   - Inferior vena cava

- Main pulmonary artery (pulmonary trunk)
- Intrapericardial portions of the right and left pulmonary artery
- Intrapericardial portions of the superior and inferior right and left pulmonary veins
  Invasion of more distal branches does not qualify for classification as T4.
5. Direct extension to parietal pericardium is classified T3 and to visceral pericardium, T4.
6. Pleural effusion is classified as T4, unless there are multiple negative cytological examinations.
7. Tumour foci in the ipsilateral parietal and visceral pleura that are discontinuous from direct pleural invasion by the primary tumour are classified T4.
8. Invasion of visceral pleura (T2) includes not only perforation of the mesothelium but also invasion of the lamina propria serosae.
9. Tumour extending to rib is classified as T3.
10. Pericardial effusion is classified the same as pleural effusion.
11. Multiple tumours of the same histological type in the same lobe is T4, but in different lobes is M1.
12. Multiple tumours of different histologic type in the same lobe or in different lobes should be classified as T1–4(m).

M Classification

Discontinuous tumours outside the parietal pleura in the chest wall or in the diaphragm are classified M1.

Small Cell Carcinoma

The TNM classification and stage grouping should be applied to small cell carcinoma. TNM is of significance for prognosis of small cell carcinoma [21], and has the advantage of providing a uniform detailed classification of tumour spread. The former categories "limited" and "extensive" for small cell carcinoma have been inconsistently defined and used.

The category "limited disease"" as used in the Veterans Administration Lung Cancer Study Group system for classification of small cell carcinoma [15] corresponds to stages I to III A and "extensive disease" to stages III B ("extensive disease I") and IV ("extensive disease II").

Bone Tumours

Summary Bone

T1	Within cortex
T2	Beyond cortex

"Skip" metastasis in the same bone as the primary is not considered in the TNM classification. Metastasis in another bone is classified as distant metastasis.

Soft Tissue Tumours

Summary Soft Tissue Sarcoma

T1	≤5 cm	
	T1a	Superficial
	T1b	Deep
T2	>5 cm	
	T2a	Superficial
	T2b	Deep

A TNM classification and stage grouping of Kaposi sarcoma are not provided. The prognosis of Kaposi sarcoma associated with AIDS is determined by AIDS.

Skin Tumours

Carcinoma of Skin

Summary Skin Carcinoma

T1	≤2 cm
T2	>2 to 5 cm
T3	>5 cm
T4	Deep extradermal structures (cartilage, skeletal muscle, bone)

1. The classification applies to any type of skin carcinoma including squamous cell, basal cell, skin appendages (e.g. sweat glands), Merkel cell.
2. The classification does not apply to carcinomas of the eyelid, vulva and penis, which have separate classifications.
3. In carcinoma of the perianal skin (anal margin), direct invasion of the mucosa or submucosa of the anal canal does not affect the T/pT classification. The tumour is classified by size.
4. Invasion of the galea aponeurotica (aponeurosis epicranialis) is classified as T4.
5. Metastastic involvement of iliac and other pelvic, abdominal or intrathoracic lymph nodes is classified as Ml.

Malignant Melanoma of Skin

Summary Malignant Melanoma

T1	≤0.75 mm	Level II
T2	>0.75 to 1.5 mm	Level III
T3	>1.5 to 4.0 mm	Level IV
T4	>4.0 mm/satellites	Level V

Rules for Classification

The classification applies to malignant melanoma of skin of all sites, including eyelid, vulva, penis and scrotum. It does not apply to melanomas arising in mucous membranes (oral cavity, nasopharynx, vagina, urethra, anal canal) or to melanomas of the conjunctiva and uvea. The last two sites have separate classifications. There is no classification for melanoma of the oral cavity, nasopharynx or other visceral sites.

pT Classification of Malignant Melanoma

Three histological criteria are considered:

- Maximum tumour thickness (Breslow) according to the largest vertical dimension of the tumour in millimetres.
  Maximum thickness of the tumour is measured with an ocular micrometer after embedding in paraffin at right angles to the adjacent normal skin. The upper reference point is the top of the granular cell layer of the epidermis of the overlying skin or the base of the ulcer if the tumour is ulcerated. The lower reference point is usually the deepest point of invasion. It may be the invading edge of a single tumour mass or an isolated cell or group of cells deep to the main mass. Melanoma cells within the epithelium of structures such as hair follicles and sebaceous glands of the skin are not taken into consideration.
- Clark levels.
- Absence or presence of satellites within 2 cm of the primary tumour.
  "Satellites" include tumour nests and nodules not only in the dermis but also in the subcutaneous tissue.

  The definitive pT category is based on these three criteria.
  In case of discrepancy between tumour thickness and level, the pT category is based on the less favourable finding.

N Classification

In-transit metastases with regional lymph node metastasis 3 cm or less in greatest dimension are classified N2b. For classification of sentinel lymph nodes see p. 7ff.

A completely different TNM classification and stage grouping have been proposed by the AJCC. It cannot be directly compared with the present classification because different criteria for T, N, and M are used. Comparative testing is recommended (see p. 23).

Breast Tumours

Rules for Classification

1. The classification applies to carcinomas of the male as well as of the female breast.

2. The rules for multiple simultaneous primary cancers in one breast (general rule No. 5, p. 3) do not apply to a single grossly detected tumour associated with multiple separate *microscopic* foci (satellites).
3. According to the proposals of the AJCC (Yarbro et al., see p. 38) LCIS should be dropped from Tis.

Regional Lymph Nodes

Intramammary lymph nodes are coded as axillary lymph nodes level I.

T Classification

Summary Breast

Tis		In situ
T1		≤ 2 cm
	T1mic	≤ 0.1 cm
	T1a	>0.1 to 0.5 cm
	T1b	>0.5 to 1 cm
	T1c	>1 to 2 cm
T2		>2 to 5 cm
T3		>5 cm
T4		Chest wall/skin
	T4a	Chest wall
	T4b	Skin oedema/ulceration, satellite skin nodules
	T4c	Both 4a and 4b
	T4d	Inflammatory carcinoma

1. The clinical estimation of tumour size by physical examination and mammography frequently give different results [4, 8, 23].
   Accuracy can be improved by using the following formula:

   $$\text{Size for classification} = 0.5 \times \text{physical examination size}$$
   $$+ 0.5 \times \text{mammographic size [23]}.$$

2. Only clinically/grossly detected satellite skin nodules are classified T4b (histologically detected foci are not considered).
3. Dimpling of the skin, nipple retraction, nipple involvement or other skin changes, except those in T4b and T4d, may occur in T1, T2 or T3 without affecting the classification. This also applies to microscopic invasion of the skin (dermis) without changes of T4b or T4d.
4. On mastectomy specimens oedema of the skin (T4b) may be inapparent at the time of pathological examination. Therefore, the surgeon should inform the pathologist of such a clinical finding to guarantee its consideration and to prevent pathological understaging.
5. Invasion of lymphatic vessels is not considered in the T category.
6. If there is a clinical picture of inflammatory carcinoma (cT4d), but a biopsy of the skin is negative for tumour and a measurable breast cancer is present, the pT category is based on the size of the tumour (pT1, 2, or 3).

7. Microscopic involvement of dermal lymphatic vessels by tumour without the clinical picture of inflammatory carcinoma is classified by the size of the tumour.

8. For T classification the size of a tumour in a biopsy should be added to the size of the tumour in the definitive resection specimen, if the biopsy specimen has a positive margin.

N/pN Classification

The N classification is done by the clinical and imaging methods usually applied for examination of the axilla. At the present time, special efforts are not required for evaluation of internal mammary lymph nodes (N3).

pN1 (movable nodes) and pN2 (nodes that are fixed to one another or to other structures) are differentiated by *macroscopic* findings of the pathologist during dissection of the axillary specimen.

Multiple micrometastasis in one axillary lymph node, e.g., 0.09 cm + 0.07 cm + 0.06 cm, should be added up (0.22 cm) and not be considered micrometastasis if larger than 0.2 cm.

Invasion of lymph vessels in the axillary fatty tissue is not considered in the N classification. It can be classified in the L- Lymphatic invasion classification (p. 12, TNM 5th edition).

For axillary nodal metastasis, the size of the metastasis, not the size of the lymph node, determines pN. If the size of the metastasis is unknown or not reported, then the pN subclassification should not be used.

For sentinel lymph nodes see p. 7ff

Gynaecological Tumours

Vulva

Summary Vulva

T1		Confined to vulva/perineum, ≤2 cm
	T1a	Stromal invasion ≤1.0 mm
	T1b	Stromal invasion >1.0 mm
T2		Confined to vulva/perineum, >2 cm
T3		Lower urethra/vagina/anus
T4		Bladder mucosa/rectal mucosa/upper urethral mucosa/bone

Invasion of the rectal wall or bladder wall (not mucosa) is classified as T3. Mucosal involvement is T4.

Invasion of the wall (not mucosa) of the upper and lower urethra is classified as T3.

Invasion of the mucosa: Lower urethra   T3
Invasion of the mucosa: Upper urethra   T4

Upper urethra corresponds to the proximal half, lower urethra to the distal half.

Vagina

Summary Vagina

T1	Vaginal wall
T2	Paravaginal tissue
T3	Extends to pelvic wall
T4	Mucosa of bladder/rectum, beyond pelvis
N1	Upper two thirds of vagina: pelvic lymph nodes
	Lower third of vagina: inguinal lymph nodes

"Frozen pelvis" is a clinical term which means that tumour extends to the pelvic wall(s). It is classified as T3.

Invasion of the rectal wall or bladder wall (not mucosa) is classified as T2. Mucosal involvement is T4.

A tumour of the upper two thirds of the vagina with inguinal lymph node metastases, is classified as M1 (Stage IV).

A tumour of the lower third of the vagina with pelvic lymph node metastasis is classified M1 (Stage IV).

Cervix Uteri

Summary Cervix Uteri

TNM				FIGO		
Tis			In situ	0		
T1			Confined to uterus	I		
	T1a		Diagnosed only by microscopy		IA	
		T1a1	Depth ≤3 mm, horizontal spread ≤7 mm			IA1
		T1a2	Depth 3–5 mm, horizontal spread ≤7 mm			IA2
	T1b		Clinically visible, greater than T1a2		IB	
		T1b1	≤4 cm			IB1
		T1b2	>4 cm			IB2
T2			Beyond uterus but not pelvic wall or lower third vagina	II		
	T2a		No parametrium		IIA	
	T2b		Parametrium		IIB	
T3			Lower third vagina/pelvic wall/ hydronephrosis	III		
	T3a		Lower third vagina		IIIA	
	T3b		Pelvic wall/hydronephrosis		IIIB	
T4			Mucosa of bladder/rectum/ beyond true pelvis	IVA		
M1			Distant metastasis	IVB		

The FIGO stages are based on clinical staging. TNM categories are based on clinical and/or pathological classification.

In the rare multifocal T1a tumours for the horizontal spread FIGO classifies by the largest focus. This is in accordance with TNM rule No. 5.

The presence of tumour cells in lymphatics (lymph vessels) or veins of the parametrium does not qualify for T2b. T2b is used only for grossly or histologically evident continuous invasion beyond the myometrium.

"Frozen pelvis" is a clinical term which means that tumour extends to the pelvic wall(s), i.e., T3b.

Invasion of the rectal wall or bladder wall (not mucosa) is classified as T3a. Mucosal involvement is T4.

Microscopic lesion greater than T1a2 (FIGO IA2) is classified as T1b1 (FIGO IB1).

Tumour-positive peritoneal fluid, e.g., in the pouch of Douglas, is not considered in the TNM or FIGO classification but should be documented.

Corpus Uteri

Summary Corpus Uteri

TNM			FIGO
Tis		In situ	0
T1		Confined to corpus	I
	T1a	Tumour limited to the endometrium	IA
	T1b	≤ 1/2 myometrium	IB
	T1c	> 1/2 myometrium	IC
T2		Extension to cervix	II
	T2a	Endocervical glandular only	IIA
	T2b	Cervical stroma	IIB
T3 and/or N1		Local and/or regional as specified below	III
	T3a	Serosa/adnexa/positive peritoneal cytology	IIIA
	T3b	Vaginal involvement	IIIB
	N1	Regional lymph node metastasis	IIIC
	T4	Mucosa of bladder/bowel	IVA
M1		Distant metastasis	IVB

T1b is "invades up to or less than one half of myometrium" (FIGO IB "invasion less than half of the myometrium").

T3a or FIGO IIIA includes discontinuous involvement of adnexae or serosa within the pelvis. Invasion of parametria is classified as T3a (FIGO IIIA).

Invasion of the rectal wall or bladder wall (not mucosa) is classified as T3b. Mucosal involvement is T4.

"Frozen pelvis" is a clinical term which means that tumour extends to the pelvic wall(s), i.e., T3b.

There may be a small number of patients with T1 corpus carcinoma who will be treated primarily with radiation therapy. For these cases FIGO recommends clinical classification according to the former FIGO schedule (IA, uterine cavity ≤8 cm in length; IB, uterine cavity >8 cm in length); the use of this staging system must be stated.

Grading

Further notes about grading appeared in the 23rd Annual Report of the FIGO [7].

Ovary

The classification applies to malignant surface epithelial-stromal tumours including those of borderline malignancy or of low malignant potential (WHO Classification, 2nd edition, Scully 1999 [26]) (corresponding to "common epithelial tumours" according to the terminology of the first edition of the WHO classification [7,25]).

Cases should be separated by histologic type and borderline or invasive nature.

The FIGO stages are based on surgical staging. TNM stages are based on clinical and/or pathological classification.

T Classification

Summary Ovary

TNM			FIGO	
T1		Limited to the ovaries	I	
	T1a	One ovary, capsule intact		IA
	T1b	Both ovaries, capsule intact		IB
	T1c	Capsule ruptured, tumour on surface, malignant cells in ascites or peritoneal washing		IC
T2		Pelvic extension	II	
	T2a	Uterus, tube(s)		IIA
	T2b	Other pelvic tissues		IIB
	T2c	Malignant cells in ascites or peritoneal washings		IIC
T3 and/or N1		Peritoneal metastasis beyond pelvis and/or regional lymph node metastasis	III	
	T3a	Microscopic peritoneal metastasis		IIIA
	T3b	Macroscopic peritoneal metastasis ≤2 cm		IIIB
	T3c and/ or N1	Peritoneal metastasis >2 cm and/ or regional lymph node metastasis		IIIC
M1		Distant metastasis (excludes peritoneal metastasis)	IV	

Tlc   Rupture of the capsule includes spontaneous rupture as well as rupture caused
by the surgeon.

T2,3   The "pelvis" includes the true or minor or small as well as the false major or
large or false pelvis.

T3   Peritoneal metastasis outside the pelvis includes involvement of the omentum.
T3 includes multifocal involvement of the peritoneum in borderline tumours.

In case of peritoneal metastasis the greatest horizontal diameter is considered in classification, not the thickness of metastasis.

Microscopic confirmation of a single peritoneal metastasis outside the pelvis, irrespective of the size of the metastasis, is required for T3. For the subdivision, size alone is relevant. Therefore, T3c is appropriate based on the macroscopic assessment by the surgeon even if microscopic confirmation was of a smaller metastasis only.

Primary extraovarian peritoneal carcinoma with or without ovarian involvement is not classified by TNM.

N Classification

Involvement of lymph nodes draining a peritoneal metastasis (T3) (e.g., mesocolic) can be considered regional lymph node metastasis (N1) rather than distant metastasis (M1).

M Classification

In ovary, peritoneal metastasis is not considered distant metastasis, it is classified as T3.

Fallopian Tube

Rules for ovary apply to fallopian tube.

Gestational Trophoblastic Tumours

Histopathological grading is not applicable.

Risk Factors Affecting Staging Include the Following

1. Urinary hCG >100,000 mIU/ml or *serum* -hCG >40,000 mIU/ml)
2. Detection of disease >6 months from termination of antecedent pregnancy

Serum hCG could be used as well as urinary hCG.
The following factors should be considered and noted in reporting:

1. Prior chemotherapy for known gestational trophoblastic disease
2. Placental site tumours should be reported separately
3. Histological verification of the disease is not required, if the hCG is abnormally elevated

Urological Tumours

Penis

Erythroplasia of Queyrat is classified as carcinoma in situ (Tis).

Prostate

T Classification

Summary Prostate

T1		Not palpable or visible
	T1a	$\leq 5\%$
	T1b	$>5\%$
	T1c	Needle biopsy
T2		Confined within prostate
	T2a	One lobe (Unilateral)*
	T2b	Both lobes (Bilateral)*
T3		Through prostatic capsule
	T3a	Extracapsular
	T3b	Seminal vesicle(s)
T4		Fixed or invades adjacent structures: bladder neck, external sphincter, rectum, levator muscles, pelvic wall

*Note. The prostate includes a right lobe, a left lobe, and a middle lobe according to the anatomic nomenclature. Therefore "unilateral" and "bilateral" are equivalent to "one lobe" and "both lobes". Involvement of the lateral lobe and the middle lobe can be considered T2a (according to TNM rule No. 4).

The prostate capsule is a network of smooth muscle and collagen-rich soft tissue around the prostate. There is no clear fascia.

There is no pT1 category because there is insufficient tissue to assess the highest pT category.

The presence of fatty or skeletal muscle tissue in a needle biopsy is not in itself evidence of invasion through the capsule into adjacent fatty tissue and thus may not be classified as T3.

Prostate carcinoma with invasion of M. sphincter urethrae internus is classified as T4.

According to newer anatomical results there are two sphincters:

M.sphincter urethrae externus = M. sphincter urethrae (diaphragmaticae)
M.sphincter urethrae internus = M. sphincter vesicae

The invasion of the M.sphincter urethrae as well as the invasion of the M.sphincter vesicae would be equivalent to an invasion of the bladder neck and should be classified as T4.

When a tumour is an incidental finding in transurethral resection (TUR) and after the first TUR a repeated TUR (re-TUR) is performed within 2 months

as part of the definitive primary treatment (without following radical prostatectomy), the subdivision into Tla and Tlb should be based on the findings of both
TURS.

Examples

1. First TUR: <5% of tissue resected involved by carcinoma. re-TUR with the same amount of
   tissue: 10% of tissue involved. Classify Tlb.
2. First TUR: 10% of tissue resected involved by carcinoma. re-TUR including a threefold amount
   of tissue: no further tumour found. Classify Tla.

Transitional cell carcinoma of the prostate (prostatic urethra) is classified
under urethra, see p. 192 of TNM 5th edition [30].

If a prostate resection specimen is limited to the prostate and does not
include the capsule or parts of the capsule (in the apex region), the pT classification cannot be used unless the tumour is clearly surrounded by nontumourous
prostate tissue.

Involvement of the prostatic urethra is not considered in the T classification.

"Frozen pelvis" is a clinical term which means that tumour extends to the
pelvic wall(s) and is fixed. It is classified as T4.

Histopathological Grading

The Gleason score and Gleason pattern [9] correspond to the grading recommended here as follows:

Gleason score	Gleason pattern	TNM histopathological grade
2–4	1,2	1
5–7	3	2
8–10	4,5	3–4

Testis

pT Classification

Summary Testis

pTis	Intratubular
pT1	Testis and epididymis, no vascular/lymphatic invasion
pT2	Testis and epididymis with vascular/lymphatic invasion or tunica vaginalis
pT3	Spermatic cord
pT4	Scrotum

In case of mixed germ cell tumours, the pT classification is determined by
the total tumour. The different components should not be classified separately.

Synchronous bilateral tumours should be staged separately as independent
primary tumours.

pT2: Invasion beyond the tunica albuginea includes invasion of any of the following — cremaster muscle, cremaster fascia, testicular portion of the internal or external spermatic fascia, i.e., invasion of the scrotum without the skin. Invasion beyond these structures into the subcutis or cutis of the scrotum is classified as pT4.

pT3: Invasion of the spermatic cord refers to direct extension.

Invasion of lymph vessels or blood vessels means unequivocal vessels lined by an endothelium.

The plexus pampiniformis belongs to the spermatic cord, so invasion should be classified as pT3.

Invasion of spermatic cord can be diagnosed, if tumour is found beyond rete testis and/or epididymis on horizontal cross sections.

Kidney

T Classification

Summary Kidney

T1	≤7.0 cm; limited to kidney
T2	>7.0 cm; limited to kidney
T3	Into major veins; adrenal or perinephric invasion
T4	Invades beyond Gerota fascia

Invasion of ipsilateral adrenal gland (T3a) refers to direct invasion.
Invasion of "perinephric tissues" (T3a) includes perirenal fat and/or renal sinus (peripelvic) fat [11].

Involvement of the renal vein (T3b) entails tumour grossly extending into the renal vein or its segmental (muscle-containing) branches, or vena cava below diaphragm [11].

Gross invasion of the wall of the vena cava above diaphragm is T3c [11].

Gerota fascia (renal fascia) includes the pre- and retrorenal fascia. Invasion of the peritoneum is invasion beyond the Gerota fascia (prerenal fascia) and is classified as T4.

Bulging of a tumour in the sense of changing the contour of the kidney is not sufficient to be classified as T3 or pT3. Penetration of the kidney capsule is needed to classify as T3 or pT3, which should be particularly searched for in the peripelvic fatty tissue.

For an optional division of T1, which is of particular interest for selection of patients for partial nephrectomy, see Chapter 5, p. 125.

Invasion (direct spread) of the contralateral adrenal gland is extremely rare and should be classified as M1.

Renal Pelvis and Ureter

Summary Renal Pelvis, Ureter

Ta	Noninvasive papillary
Tis	In situ
T1	Subepithelial connective tissue
T2	Muscularis
T3	Beyond muscularis
T4	Adjacent organs, perinephric fat

1. Direct extension into the urinary bladder in the region of the ostium is classified by the depth of greatest invasion in any of the involved organs.
2. In tumours of the ureter, adjacent organs include parietal peritoneum.
3. The prognosis of T3 in ureter is worse than in renal pelvis and corresponds approximately to T4 renal pelvis tumours. Therefore, separate analysis of ureter and renal pelvis carcinoma is recommended [10].
4. For classification of multiple synchronous primary tumours renal pelvis and ureter are considered a single organ. Therefore, in cases of synchronous tumours in the renal pelvis and the ureter, the tumour with the highest T category should be classified and the multiplicity or the number of tumours should be indicated in parentheses, e. g., T2(m) or T3(2). In case of multifocal tumours of renal pelvis and ureter with Ta and Tis tumours, Tis(m) should be classified. In contrast, in case of synchronous tumours in the renal pelvis and the urinary bladder both tumours should be classified independently.

Urinary Bladder

The classification applies not only to carcinomas (noninvasive or invasive) but also to the newly introduced "Papillary urothelial (transitional cell) neoplasm of low malignant potential."*

Summary Urinary Bladder

Ta		Noninvasive papillary
Tis		In situ: flat tumour
T1		Subepithelial connective tissue
T2		Muscularis
	T2a	Inner half
	T2b	Outer half
T3		Beyond muscularis
	T3a	Microscopically
	T3b	Extravesical mass

---

* Mostofi FK, Davis CJ, Sesterhenn IA (eds) Histological Typing of Bladder Tumours. 2nd ed. (World Health Organization [WHO] International Histological Classification of Tumours). Springer: Berlin Heidelberg New York, 1999

T4		Prostate, uterus, vagina, pelvic wall, abdominal wall
	T4a	Prostate, uterus, vagina
	T4b	Pelvic wall, abdominal wall

1. In case of multifocal tumours of urinary bladder with Ta and Tis tumours, Tis(m) should be classified.
2. If the pathology specimen does not contain muscle, the category T1 is applicable (see TNM Classification 1997 [30], General rule No. 4). However, the pathology report should state the absence of muscle to allow the clinician to consider repeating the biopsy.
3. In case of transurethral resection, differentiation between T2a and T2b is possible only if the surgeon submits the material as superficial (inner) and deep (outer) portions and histological examination is performed separately. Otherwise, the case is classified as T2.
4. In some cases (up to 50%) a lamina muscularis mucosae has been described. Invasion of muscularis means lamina muscularis propria.
5. Direct invasion of the distal ureter is classified by the depth of greatest invasion in any of the involved organs.
6. Uncommonly, carcinomas of the bladder show an associated in situ component extending into the prostatic ducts and sometimes into the prostatic glands (or ureter) without any invasion in the prostate. Such cases are classified according to the depth of bladder wall invasion. The extension of the associated in situ component into the prostate does not qualify for classification as T4. It may be indicated by the suffix "(is)", e. g., T2(is). It may be further indicated by the suffix "(is pu)"(extension into the prostatic urethra) or "(is pd)"(extension into the prostatic ducts), e. g., T2(is pu) or T2 (is pd).
7. Invasion of prostatic urethra (extension of invasive urinary bladder carcinoma into the prostatic urethra with invasion of the latter) is included in prostatic invasion and therefore classified as T4a.
8. Direct invasion of the large or small intestine should be classified as T4a. The same applies to invasion through the peritoneum covering the bladder.
9. Invasion of seminal vesicles by bladder tumours should be classified as T4a.

Recurrent Carcinoma After Cystectomy and Ureterosigmoidostomy

A recurrent transitional carcinoma in the region of a ureterosigmoidostomy may invade only the subepithelial connective tissue of the ureter and the adjacent mucosa and submucosa of the sigmoid colon. In this case, the invasion of the colon should not be considered as invasion of an adjacent organ. For the T classification the rules for ureter and colon should be applied, i.e., rT1 is the correct classification.

Urethra

T Classification

Summary Urethra

Ta	Noninvasive papillary, polypoid, or verrucous
Tis	In situ
T1	Subepithelial connective Tissue
T2	Corpus spongiosum, prostate, periurethral muscle
T3	Corpus cavernosum, beyond prostatic capsule anterior vagina, bladder neck
T4	Other adjacent organs

In urethral diverticular carcinoma, a differentiation between T2 and T3 is not possible [3]. In this case T2 is used (according to TNM rule No. 4).

Ophthalmic Tumours

Carcinoma of Eyelid

The eyelids are covered externally by epidermis (anterior surface of the eyelid) and internally by conjunctiva (posterior surface). This classification applies only to the carcinomas of the anterior surface of the eyelid and the eyelid margin. Carcinomas of the posterior surface of the eyelid are considered under tumours of the conjunctiva.

Carcinoma of Conjunctiva

This classification applies to carcinoma of the palpebral and bulbar conjunctiva and the conjunctival fornix.

Malignant Melanoma of Conjunctiva

This classification applies to malignant melanoma of the palpebral and bulbar conjunctiva and the conjunctival fornix.

Involvement of eyelid is defined as invasion beyond the tarsal plate into the anterior part of the eyelid.

Sarcoma of Orbit

In tumours of the orbital soft tissues T3 is used for those with *diffuse* invasion of the orbit and/or with invasion of the bony walls. In tumours of the orbital bones T3 is used for invasion of the orbital soft tissues.

Hodgkin and Non-Hodgkin Lymphomas

Right or left neck are separate lymph node regions.

1. Single lymph node regions are:
   - Lymph nodes of head, face and neck
   - Intrathoracic lymph nodes

- Intra-abdominal lymph nodes
- Lymph nodes of axilla or arm
- Lymph nodes of inguinal region or leg
- Pelvic lymph nodes

Bilateral involvement of axilla/arm lymph nodes is considered as involvement of two separate regions. The same applies to bilateral involvement of inguinal lymph nodes.

Examples

Involvement	Classification
Parotid and jugular	Single node region
Jugular and tracheal	Two regions, same side of diaphragm
Tracheal, hilar, para-aortic abdominal	Two regions, both sides of diaphragm
Axillary, bilateral	Two regions, same side of diaphragm
Inguinal bilateral	Two regions, same side of diaphragm

2. Direct spread of a lymphoma into adjacent tissues or organs does not influence classification.

Examples
   - Lymphoma of a cervical lymph node with pericapsular extension into adjacent muscle — stage I
   - Gastric lymphoma with direct spread to pancreas and involvement of perigastric lymph nodes — stage IIE
   - Lymphoma involving the ascending colon, caecum and ileocaecal valve with direct extension to the terminal ileum — stage IE

3. Involvement of two or more segments of the gastrointestinal tract, isolated and not in continuity, is classified as stage IV (disseminated involvement of one or more extralymphatic organs).
   Example. Involvement of stomach and of ileum — stage IV.

4. For classification of extranodal lymphomas, involvement of both organs of a paired site is considered as involvement of a single organ.
   Example. Extranodal lymphoma involving both lungs is classified stage IE.

5. Multifocal involvement of a single extralymphatic organ is classified stage IE and not stage IV.

6. Primary Extranodal Lymphomas, Stage IIE: The definitions of regional lymph nodes given for the individual tumour sites apply to extranodal lymphomas, too, e. g., for primary gastric lymphomas the regional lymph nodes are the perigastric nodes along the lesser and greater curvatures and the nodes located along the left gastric, common hepatic, splenic and coeliac arteries.

For further explanatory notes see p. 34ff.

Appendix

Comparison of the regional lymph nodes listed in the UICC [30] and the AJCC TNM 5th editions [1]

SITE	UICC	AJCC
Lip and oral cavity	Cervical	
		Submental
		Submandibular
		Jugular, upper, mid, lower
		Posterior triangle (spinal accessory) upper, lower
		Prelaryngeal (Delphian)
		Pretracheal
		Paratracheal
		Upper mediastinal
		Buccinator (facial)
		Intraparotid
		Preauricular
		Postauricular
		Suboccipital
Pharynx	Cervical	
		Submental
		Submandibular
		Jugular, upper, mid, lower
		Posterior triangle (spinal accessory) upper, lower
		Prelaryngeal (Delphian)
		Pretracheal
		Paratracheal
		Upper mediastinal
		Buccinator (facial)
		Intraparotid
		Preauricular
		Postauricular
Larynx	Cervical	
		Submental
		Submandibular
		Jugular, upper, mid, lower
		Posterior triangle (spinal accessory) upper, lower

SITE	UICC	AJCC
		Prelaryngeal (Delphian)
		Pretracheal
		Paratracheal
		Upper mediastinal
		Buccinator (facial)
		Intraparotid
		Preauricular
		Postauricular
		Suboccipital
Paranasal sinuses	Cervical	
		Submental
		Submandibular
		Jugular, upper, mid, lower
		Posterior triangle (spinal accessory) upper, lower
		Prelaryngeal (Delphian)
		Pretracheal
		Paratracheal
		Upper mediastinal
		Buccinator (facial)
		Intraparotid
		Preauricular
		Postauricular
		Suboccipital
Salivary glands	Cervical	
		Submental
		Submandibular
		Jugular, upper, mid, lower
		Posterior triangle (spinal accessory) upper, lower
		Prelaryngeal (Delphian)
		Pretracheal
		Paratracheal
		Upper mediastinal
		Buccinator (facial)
		Intraparotid
		Preauricular
		Postauricular
		Suboccipital
Thyroid	Cervical	
		Suboccipital
		Submandibular
		Jugular, upper, mid, lower

SITE	UICC	AJCC
		Posterior triangle (spinal accessory) upper, lower
		Prelaryngeal (Delphian)
		Pretracheal
		Paratracheal
	Upper mediastinal	Upper mediastinal
		Buccinator (facial)
		Intraparotid
		Preauricular
		Postauricular
		Suboccipital
Cervical oesophagus	Cervical, including supraclavicular	Scalene
		Internal jugular
		Upper cervical
		Perioesophageal
		Supraclavicular
		Cervical, NOS
Intrathoracic oesophagus, upper, middle, lower	Mediastinal Perigastric (excluding celiac)	Tracheobronchial
		Superior mediastinal
		Peritracheal
		Carinal
		Hilar (pulmonary roots)
		Perioesophageal
		Perigastric
		Paracardial
		Mediastinal NOS
Stomach	Perigastric along lesser and greater curvatures	Perigastric along lesser and greater curvatures
	Nodes along left gastric, common hepatic, splenic, and celiac arteries	Nodes along left gastric, common hepatic, splenic, and celiac arteries
		Greater Curvature of Stomach:
		Greater curvature
		Greater omental
		Gastroduodenal
		Gastroepiploic, rights or NOS
		Gastroepiploic, left
		Pyloric, including subpyloric and infra pyloric

SITE	UICC	AJCC
		Pancreaticoduodenal (anteriorly along first part of the duodenum)
		Pancreatic and splenic area: Pancreaticolienal Peripancreatic Splenic hilum
		Lesser curvature of Stomach: Lesser curvature Lesser omental Left gastric Paracardial; cardial Cardioesophageal Perigastic, NOS Common hepatic Celiac Hepatoduodenal
		All other lymph nodes are considered distant. They include: Retropancreatic Para-aortic Portal Retroperitoneal Mesenteric
Small intestine, duodenum	Pancreaticoduodenal Pyloric Hepatic (pericholedochal, cystic, hilar) Superior mesenteric	Duodenal Hepatic Pancreaticoduodenal Infrapyloric Gastroduodenal Pyloric Superior mesenteric Pericholedochal Regional lymph nodes, NOS
Small intestine, ileum and jejunum	Mesenteric nodes, Superior mesenteric Ileocolic (terminal ileum only) Mesenteric, NOS	Posterior cecal (terminal ileum only) Ileocolic (terminal ileum only) Superior mesenteric Mesenteric, NOS Regional lymph nodes, NOS

SITE	UICC	AJCC
Cecum and appendix	Nodes along the ileocolic, and right colic arteries	Anterior cecal Posterior cecal Ileocolic Right colic
Ascending colon	Nodes along the ileocolic, right colic, and middle colic arteries	Ileocolic Right colic Middle colic
Colon Hepatic flexure	Nodes along the right colic, and middle colic arteries	Middle colic Right colic
Transverse colon	Nodes along the right colic, middle colic, and left colic arteries and inferior mesenteric	Middle colic
Colon Splenic flexure	Nodes along the middle colic, left colic, and inferior mesenteric arteries	Middle colic Left colic Inferior mesenteric
Descending colon	Nodes along the left colic, inferior mesenteric	Left colic Inferior mesenteric Superior rectal (hemorrhoidal) Sigmoidal Sigmoid mesenteric
Sigmoid colon	Sigmoid nodes, left colic Nodes along the inferior mesenteric, and superior rectal arteries	Inferior mesenteric Superior rectal (hemorrhoidal) Sigmoidal Sigmoid mesenteric
Colon Rectosigmoid	Sigmoid nodes, left colic node Nodes along the left colic, inferior mesenteric, and superior rectal (hemorrhoidal) arteries Pericolic, Perirectal	Perirectal Left colic Sigmoid mesenteric Sigmoidal Inferior mesenteric Superior rectal (hemorrhoidal) Middle rectal (hemorrhoidal)

SITE	UICC	AJCC
Rectum	Nodes along the superior rectal (hemorrhoidal), inferior mesenteric, and internal iliac arteries Perirectal	Perirectal Sigmoid mesenteric Inferior mesenteric Lateral, sacral, presacral Internal iliac Sacral promontory (Gerota') Superior rectal (hemorrhoidal) Middle rectal (hemorrhoidal) Inferior rectal (hemorrhoidal)
Anal canal	Perirectal Internal iliac Inguinal	Perirectal (anorectal, perirectal, lateral sacral) Internal iliac (hypogastric) Inguinal (superficial, deep femoral)
Liver	Hilar (those in the hepatoduodenal ligament)*	Hilar nodes[1] (those in the hepatoduodenal ligament) Hepatic Periportal including those along the hepatic artery, portal vein, and inferior vena cava
Gallbladder	Superior mesenteric Peripancreatic (head only) Cystic duct node Pericholedochal Hilar Celiac Periduodenal Periportal	 Cystic duct Pericholedochal Hilar Celiac Periduodenal Periportal
Extrahepatic bile ducts	Celiac Cystic duct Hilar	 Cystic Hilar

*Note that the UICC adopted the AJCC regional lymph node list in May 1999 based on studies by Nozaki et al. [22]

[1]Regional nodes include those along the hepatic artery, portal vein, and inferior vena cava.

SITE	UICC	AJCC
	Superior mesenteric Periduodenal	Superior mesenteric Periduodenal Posterior pancreaticoduodenal
	Peripancreatic (head only)	Peripancreatic
	Periportal Pericholedochal	Periportal Pericholedochal Celiac
Ampulla of Vater	Superior: Lymph nodes superior to the head and body of the pancreas. Inferior: Lymph nodes inferior to the head and body of the pancreas	Superior: Lymph nodes superior to the head and body of the pancreas Inferior: Lymph nodes inferior to the head and body of the pancreas
	Anterior: Anterior pancreaticoduodenal, pyloric and proximal mesenteric	Anterior: Anterior pancreaticoduodenal, pytonic proximal mesenteric
	Posterior: Posterior pancreaticoduodenal, common bile duct, and proximal mesenteric	Posterior: Posterior pancreatoduodenal common bite duct mesenteric lymph
		Others: Pancreaticoduodenal, NOS Peripancreatic Infrapyloric Hepatic Subpyloric Celiac Superior mesenteric Retroperitoneal Lateral aortic
Exocrine pancreas	Celiac (for tumours of head only) Superior: Lymph nodes superior to the head and body of the pancreas	Superior: Lymph nodes superior to the head and body of the pancreas

SITE	UICC	AJCC
	Inferior: Lymph nodes inferior to the head and body of the pancreas	Inferior: Lymph nodes inferior to the head and body of the pancreas
	Anterior: Anterior pancreaticoduodenal, pyloric (for the tumours of head only) and proximal mesenteric lymph nodes	Anterior: Anterior pancreaticoduodenal, proximal mesenteric lymph nodes
	Posterior: Posterior pancreaticoduodenal, common bile duct or pericholedochal and proximal mesenteric lymph nodes	Posterior: Posterior pancreaticoduodenal, bile duct or pericholedochal and proximal mesenteric lymph nodes
	Splenic: hilum of spleen and tail of pancreas (for tumours in the body and tail only)	Splenic: (for tumours in the body and tail only)
		Retroperitoneal
Vagina	Pelvic nodes (upper 2/3 of vagina)	Pelvic, NOS (upper 2/3 only)
	Inguinal nodes (lower 1/3 of vagina)	Inguinal nodes (lower 1/3 of vagina)
		Iliac, common, internal, external
		Hypogastric (obturator)
		Pelvic, NOS (upper 2/3 only)
Cervix uteri	Paracervical	Paracervical
	Parametrial	Parametrial
	Hypogastric (internal iliac obturator)	Hypogastric (obturator)
	Iliac, common and external	Common iliac
	Iliac, common and external	Common iliac
		External iliac
		Internal iliac

SITE	UICC	AJCC
	Presacral	Presacral
	Lateral sacral	Sacral
Corpus uteri	Pelvic (hypogastric [obturator, internal iliac] common	Hypogastric (obturator)
	and external iliac, parametrial, and sacral)	Internal iliac
	Para-aortic nodes	Common iliac
		External iliac
		Parametrial
		Sacral
Ovary	Hypogastric (obturator)	Hypogastric (obturator)
	Common iliac	Common iliac
	External iliac	External iliac
	Lateral sacral	Lateral sacral
	Para-aortic	Para-aortic
	Inguinal	Inguinal
		Pelvic, NOS
		Retroperitoneal, NOS
Fallopian tube	Hypogastric (obturator)	Hypogastric (obturator)
	Common iliac	Common iliac
	External iliac	External iliac
	Lateral sacral	Lateral sacral
	Para-aortic	Para-aortic
	Inguinal	Inguinal
		Internal iliac
Penis	Superficial and deep inguinal	Single superficial inguinal (femoral)
		Multiple or bilateral superficial inguinal
		Deep inguinal: Rosenmüller or Cloque
		External iliac
		Internal iliac (hypogastric)
	Pelvic nodes	Pelvic nodes, NOS
Prostate	Pelvic nodes below bifurcation of common iliac arteries	Pelvis, NOS
		Hypogastric Obturator
		Iliac (internal, external, NOS)

SITE	UICC	AJCC
		Sacral (lateral, presacral, promontory (NOS)
Testis	Abdominal para-aortic, preaortic, interaortocaval, precaval, paracaval, retrocaval, retroaortic nodes.	Interaortocaval, para-aortic, paracaval, preaortic, precaval retroaortic, retrocaval nodes.
	Nodes along the spermatic vein.	Nodes along the spermatic vein
	After scrotal or inguinal surgery: inguinal nodes.	After scrotal or inguinal surgery: intrapelvic, external iliac, inguinal nodes.
Kidney	Hilar, abdominal para-aortic, paracaval nodes.	Renal hilar, paracaval, Aortic (para-aortic, periaortic, lateral aortic), retroperitoneal, NOS
Renal Pelvis and Ureter	Hilar, addominal para-aortic, paracaval nodes. For ureter: Intrapelvic nodes.	For renal pelvis: Renal hilar, paracaval, retroperitoneal, NOS For ureter: Renal hilar, Iliac (common, internal [hypogastric], external), paracaval, peri-ureteral, pelvic, NOS
Urinary Bladder	Pelvic nodes below the bifurcation of the common iliac arteries. (Nodes of the true pelvis).	Nodes below the bifurcation of the common iliac arteries: Hypogastric, obdurator, iliac (internal, external, NOS), perivesical, pelvic, NOS, Sacral (lateral, sacral promontory [Gerota's]), Presacral
Urethra	Inguinal and pelvic nodes.	Inguinal (superficial or deep), Iliac (common, internal hypogastric], obdurator, external), presacral, Sacral, NOS, pelvic, NOS

References

[1] *AJCC Cancer staging manual.* 5th edition. Fleming ID, Cooper JS, Henson DE, Hutter RVP, Kennedy BJ, Murphy GP, O'Sullivan B, Sobin LH, Yarbro JW (eds), Lippincott, Philadelphia, 1997

[2] Alberti PW, Boyce DB (eds) *Workshops from the centennial conference on laryngeal cancer.* Appleton Century Crofts, New York, 1976

[3] Clayton M, Siami F, Guinan P. Urethral diverticular carcinoma. *Cancer* 1992; **70**: 665–670

[4] De Wolfe CJM, Perry NM (eds) *European guidelines for quality assurance in mammography screening.* (2nd ed.) European Commission, Brussels, 1996

[5] Dralle H. Personal communication, 1992

[6] Fielding LP, Arsenault PA, Chapuis PH, et al. Clinicopathological staging for colorectal cancer: an International Documentation System (IDS) and an International Comprehensive Anatomical Terminology (ICAT). *J Gastroenterol Hepatol* 1991; **6**: 325–344

[7] FIGO Annual Report on the Results on the Treatment in Gynaecological Cancer. 23rd vol. Pecorelli S, Boyle P, Odicino F, Sideri M Maisonneuve P, Severi G, Zigliani L (eds) *J Epidemiol Biostat* 1998; **3**: 1–168

[8] Fornage BD, Tonbas O, Morel M. Clinical, mammographic, and sonographic determination of preoperative breast cancer size. *Cancer* 1987; **60**: 765–771

[9] Gleason DF, Veterans Administration Cooperative Urological Research Group (VACURG) Histologic grading and clinical staging of prostatic carcinoma. In *Urologic pathology: the prostate,* Tannenbaum M (ed) Lea and Febiger: Philadelphia, 1977

[10] Guinan P, Vogelzang NJ, Randazzo R, et al. Renal pelvic transitional cell carcinoma. The role of the kidney in tumor-node-metastasis staging. *Cancer* 1992; **69**: 1773–1775

[11] Guinan P, Sobin LH, Algaba F, et al. TNM staging of renal cell carcinoma. Report of Workgroup 3. *Cancer* 1997; **80**: 992–993

[12] Goldstein NS, Turner JR. Pericolonic tumors deposits in patients with T3N+M0 colon adenocarcinomas: a marker for reduced disease-free survival and intra-abdominal metastasis. *Cancer* 2000; **88**: 2228–2238.

[13] Harrison JC, Dean PJ, El-Zeky F, Vander Zwaag R. From Dukes through Jass. Pathological prognostic indicators in rectal cancer. *Hum Pathol* 1994; **25**: 498–505

[14] Harrison JC, Dean PJ, El-Zeky F, Vander Zwaag R. Impact of the Crohn's like lymphoid reaction on staging of right-sided colon cancer. Results of a multivariate analysis. *Hum Pathol* 1995; **26**: 31–38

[15] Hyde L, Yee J, Wilson R, Patno ME. Cell type and the natural history of lung cancer. *JAMA* 1965; **193**: 52–54

[16] Jamieson JK, Dobson JF. The lymphatics of the colon. *Proc R Soc Med* 1909; **2**: 149–152

[17] Japanese Research Society for Gastric Cancer. Japanese classification of gastric carcinoma. (1st English ed.) Nishi M, Omori Y, Miwa K, (eds) Kanehara: Tokyo, 1995

[18] Japanese Gastric Cancer Association (JGCA). Japanese classification of gastric carcinoma. 2nd English edition. *Gastric Cancer* 1998; **1**: 10–24

[19] Kleinsasser O. *Tumoren des Larynx und des Hypopharynx.* Thieme: Stuttgart, 1987

[20] Kleinsasser O. Revision of classification of laryngeal cancer, is it long overdue? (Proposals for an improved TN-classification) *J Laryngol Otol* 1992; **106**: 197–204

[21] Mountain CF. Prognostic implications of the international staging system for lung. *Semin Oncol* 1988; **15**: 236–245

[22] Nozaki Y, Yamamoto M, Ikai, I, et al. Reconsideration of the lymph node metastasis pattern (N factor) from intrahepatic cholangiocarcinoma using the International Union Against Cancer TNM staging system for primary liver carcinoma. *Cancer* 1998; **83**: 1923–1929

[23] Pain JA, Ebbs SR, Hern RPA, et al. Assessment of breast cancer size: a comparison of methods. *Eur J Surg Oncol* 1992; **18**: 44–48

[24] Robbins KT, Medina JE, Wolfe GT, et al. Standardizing neck dissection terminology. Official report of the Academy Committee for Head and Neck Surgery and Oncology. *Arch Otolaryngol Head Neck Surg* 1991; **117**: 601–605

[25] Serov SF. Scully RE, Sobin LH. *Histological typing of ovarian tumours* (WHO International Histological Classification of Tumours No. 9). World Health Organization: Geneva, 1973

[26] Scully RE. *Histological typing of ovarian tumours* (2nd ed.). (WHO International Histological Classification of Tumours). Springer: Berlin Heidelberg New York, 1999

[27] Siewert JR, Stein HJ. Classification of adenocarcinoma of the esophagogastric junction. *Br J Surg* 1998; **85**: 1457–1459

[28] Siewert JR. Adenocarcinoma of the esophagogastric junction. *Gastric Cancer* 1999; **2**: 87–88

[29] Soreide O, Norstein J, Fielding LP, et al. International standardization and documentation of the treatment of rectal cancer. In: *Rectal cancer surgery*, Soreide O, Norstein J (eds). Springer: Berlin Heidelberg New York, 1997, pp. 405–455

[30] *UICC (International Union against Cancer) TNM Classification of Malignant Tumours.* (5th ed.) Sobin LH, Wittekind Ch (eds). Wiley-Liss: New York, 1997

[31] *UICC (International Union against Cancer) TNM Atlas. Illustrated Guide to the TNM/pTNM Classification of Malignant Tumours* (4th ed. 1997. Corrected second printing 1999). Hermanek P, Hutter RVP, Sobin LH, Wagner G, Wittekind Ch (eds) Springer, Berlin Heidelberg New York

[32] Zeng Z, Cohen AM, Hajdu S, et al. Serosal cytologic study to determine free mesothelial penetration by intraperitoneal colon cancer. *Cancer* 1992; **70**: 737–740

Site-Specific Recommendations for pT and pN

Introduction

This chapter is an expansion of the following general rules of the TNM system (TNM Classification 1997 [13], pp. 7, 8):

> 2b. Pathological assessment of the primary tumour (pT) entails a resection of the primary tumour or biopsy adequate to evaluate the highest pT category. The pathological assessment of the regional lymph nodes (pN) entails removal of nodes adequate to validate the absence of regional lymph node metastasis (pN0) and sufficient to evaluate the highest pN category.
> 4. If there is doubt concerning the correct T, N or M category to which a particular case should be allotted, then the lower (i.e., less advanced) category should be chosen.

In the TNM Classification of 1997 [13] these general rules have been specified for breast cancer only. Analogous definitions for the pN0 category of other tumour sites are given in the 1997 TNM Classification, except for bone, soft tissues, urological, and ophthalmic tumours.

The numbers of lymph nodes given in the different tumour sites are considered adequate for staging. If the examined lymph nodes are negative but the number ordinarily resected is not met, classify as pN0. The number of nodes examined and the number involved by tumour should be recorded in the pathology report [1, 2, 4, 6, 7, 9]. This information may also be added in parentheses, e.g., for colorectal carcinoma pN0 (0/11) or pN1 (3/10).

In many tumour sites, the number of involved regional lymph nodes indicates differences in prognosis. For details, see p. 75. A correlation exists between the number of examined lymph nodes and the pN classification. With increasing number of examined lymph nodes a higher frequency of lymph node-positive cases is found and-in tumour sites where more than one positive pN category is provided-a greater proportion of higher pN categories can be observed [3, 11].

Therefore, the number of examined lymph nodes reflects the reliability of the pN classification.

Head and Neck Tumours

pT–Primary Tumour

Site	pT3 or less *Recommendation for all sites*	pT4 *Microscopic confirmation of:*
Lip	Pathological examination of the primary carcinoma with *no gross tumour at* the margins of resection (with or without microscopic involvement)	Invasion of adjacent structures, e.g., spongious bone, tongue or skin of neck
Oral Cavity		Invasion of adjacent structures, e.g., spongious bone, deep (extrinsic) muscle of tongue, maxillary sinus or skin.
Oropharynx		Invasion of adjacent structures, e.g., plerygoid muscle(s), mandible, hard palate or deep (extrinsic) muscle of tongue.
Nasopharynx		Invasion of cranial nerves, infratemporal fossa, orbit, hypopharynx or intracranial extension.
Hypopharynx		Invasion of adjacent structures, e.g., thyroid/cricoid cartilage, carotid artery, soft tissues of neck, prevertebral fascia/muscles, thyroid,and/or oesophagus.
Larynx		Invasion of tissue beyond the larynx, e.g., on the outer side of thyroid or cricoid cartilage, oesophagus or soft tissues of neck.
Maxillary Sinus		Invasion of the orbital contents beyond the floor or medial wall including any of the following: the orbital apex, cribriform plate, base of skull, nasopharynx, sphenoid, frontal sinuses.

Site	pT3 or less *Recommendation for all sites*	pT4 *Microscopic confirmation of:*
Ethmoid sinus		Intracranial extension, orbital extension including apex, involvement of sphenoid and/or frontal sinus, and/or skin of nose.
Salivary Glands		Invasion of base of the skull, seventh cranial nerve, and/or size >6 cm in greatest dimension.
Thyroid Gland		Invasion of tissue beyond the thyroid capsule.

pN–Regional Lymph Nodes

The site-specific recommendations regarding number of nodes for diagnosis of pN0 for all sites of head and neck tumours have been incorporated in the 5th edition [13] (see Table 3).

Site	Recommendations
All sites except thyroid gland and nasopharynx	**pN1** Microscopic confirmation of metastasis in a single ipsilateral lymph node, 3 cm or less in greatest dimension **pN2** Microscopic confirmation of a regional lymph node metastasis more than 3 cm but not more than 6 cm in greatest dimension *or* microscopic confirmation of at least two regional lymph node metastases, none more than 6 cm in greatest dimension **pN3** Microscopic confirmation of a regional lymph node metastasis more than 6 cm in greatest dimension

Notes. 1. Terminology of neck dissection [8]: A radical neck dissection includes the removal of all ipsilateral cervical lymph node groups, i.e., lymph nodes from levels I through V (see p. 25ff) and removal of the spinal accessory nerve, internal jugular vein and sternocleidomastoid muscle.

In a modified radical neck dissection the same lymph nodes are removed as in a radical neck dissection; however, one or more nonlymphatic structures are preserved.

A selective neck dissection is a neck dissection with preservation of one or more lymph node groups routinely removed in radical neck dissection.

The most often performed types of selective neck dissections are: (a) supraomohyoid dissection, levels I–III; (b) posterolateral neck dissection, levels II–V and the retroauricular and occipital (suboccipital) nodes; (c) lateral neck dissection, levels II–IV, (d) anterior compartment neck dissection, level VI.

Table 3. Number of lymph nodes usually examined in lymph node dissection specimens to classify pN0

Site	Number of lymph nodes usually examined in lymph node dissection specimens to classify pN0	
Lip and oral cavity	6	Selective neck dissection specimen
	10	Radical or modified radical neck dissection specimen
Pharynx	6	Selective neck dissection specimen
	10	Radical or modified radical neck dissection specimen
Larynx	6	Selective neck dissection specimen
	10	Radical or modified radical neck dissection specimen
Paranasal sinuses	6	Selective neck dissection specimen
	10	Radical or modified radical neck dissection specimen
Salivary glands	6	Selective neck dissection specimen
	10	Radical or modified radical neck dissection specimen
Thyroid gland	6	
Oesophagus	6	
Stomach	15	
Small intestine	6	
Colon and rectum	12	
Anal canal	12	Perirectal-pelvic lymphadenectomy specimen
	6	Inguinal lymphadenectomy specimen
Liver	3	
Gallbladder	3	
Extrahepatic bile ducts	3	
Ampulla of Vater	10	
Pancreas	10	
Lung	6	
Bone and soft tissues	—	
Carcinoma of the skin	6	
Malignant melanoma of skin	6	
Breast	6	
Vulva	6	
Vagina	6	Inguinal lymphadenectomy specimen
	10	Pelvic lymphadenectomy specimen
Cervix uteri	10	
Corpus uteri	10	
Ovary	10	
Fallopian tube	10	
Penis	6	
Prostate	8	
Testis	8	
Kidney	8	
Renal pelvis and ureter	8	
Urinary bladder	8	
Urethra	8	
Ophthalmic tumours	6	
All sites and types		

2. If the size of a *biopsied* lymph node is not indicated by the submitting surgeon, classify pN1 if the positive biopsy is from one node and pN2 if positive biopsies are from two or more lymph nodes.

Nasopharynx

pN1

Microscopic confirmation of unilateral metastasis in lymph node(s), 6 cm or less in greatest dimension, above supraclavicular fossa

pN2

Microscopic confirmation of bilateral metastasis in lymph node(s), 6 cm or less in greatest dimension, above supraclavicular fossa

pN3

Microscopic confirmation of metastasis in lymph node(s)
a) greater than 6 cm in dimension
b) in the supraclavicular fossa

Thyroid Gland

pN1a

Microscopic confirmation of a metastasis in an ipsilateral cervical lymph node

pN1b

Microscopic confirmation of a midline or contralateral cervical or mediastinal lymph node metastasis

Digestive System Tumours

pT–Primary Tumour

Site	Recommendations
Oesophagus	**pT3 or less** Pathological examination of the primary carcinoma with *no gross tumour* at the deep (radial, lateral), proximal and distal margins of the resection (with or without microscopic involvement)
	pT4 Microscopic confirmation of invasion of adjacent structures

Stomach

pT3 or less
Pathological examination of the primary carcinoma removed by total or partial gastrectomy with *no gross tumour* at the deep (radial, lateral), proximal and distal margins of resection (with or without microscopic involvement) *or* Pathological examination of the primary carcinoma removed by endoscopic polypectomy or local excision with histologically tumour-free margins of resection

pT4
Microscopic confirmation of invasion of adjacent structures such as spleen, transverse colon, liver, diaphragm, pancreas, abdominal wall, adrenal gland, kidney, small intestine and/or retroperitoneum

Small
Intestine

pT3 or less
Pathological examination of the primary carcinoma removed by short segment (limited) or radical resection with *no gross tumour* at the deep (radial, lateral), proximal and distal margins of resection (with or without microscopic involvement) *or* Pathological examination of the primary carcinoma removed by endoscopic polypectomy or local excision with histologically tumour-free margins of resection

pT4
Pathological confirmation of perforation of the visceral peritoneum *or* Microscopic confirmation of invasion of other organs or structures (including other loops of small intestine, mesentery or retroperitoneum more than 2 cm and abdominal wall via serosa; for duodenum only, invasion of pancreas)

Colon and Rectum

pT3 or less
Pathological examination[1] of the primary carcinoma removed by short segment (limited) or radical resection with *no gross tumour* at the deep (radial, lateral, circumferential), proximal and distal margins of resection (with or without microscopic involvement) *or* Pathological examination of the primary carcinoma removed by endoscopic polypectomy or local excision with histologically tumour-free margins of resection

[1]**Note.** Pathological confirmation may be achieved from biopsies or resection specimens or by cytology of specimens obtained from the serosa overlying the primary tumour [14].

pT4
Pathological confirmation of perforation of the visceral peritoneum *or* Microscopic confirmation of invasion of adjacent organs or structures (including invasion of levator muscles) and invasion of other segments of the colorectum by way of the sorosa

Anal Canal

pT3 or less
Pathological examination of the primary carcinoma with *no gross tumour* at the margins of resection (with or without microscopic involvement)

pT4
Microscopic confirmation of invasion of adjacent organs (e.g. vagina, urethra, bladder) [invasion of the sphincter muscle(s) alone is not sufficient for pT4]

Liver

pT3 or less
Pathological examination of the primary carcinoma with *no gross tumour* at the margins of resection (with or without microscopic involvement)

pT4
Microscopic confirmation of multiple tumours in more than one lobe *or* Microscopic confirmation of invasion of a major branch of the portal or hepatic vein(s) or tumour(s) with direct invasion of adjacent organ(s) other than gallbladder, or tumour(s) with perforation of the visceral peritoneum

Gallbladder

pT3 or less
Pathological examination of the primary carcinoma with *no gross tumour* at the margins of resection (with or without microscopic involvement)

pT4
Microscopic confirmation of tumour in the liver more than 2 cm from the gallbladder or invasion of at least two adjacent organs (stomach, duodenum, colon, pancreas, omentum, extrahepatic bile ducts, liver)

Extrahepatic Bile Ducts

pT2 or less
Pathological examination of the primary carcinoma with *no gross tumour* at the margins of resection (with or without microscopic involvement)

pT3
Microscopic confirmation of invasion of adjacent structures (liver, pancreas, duodenum, gallbladder, colon, stomach)

Ampulla of Vater **pT3 or less**
Pathological examination of the primary carcinoma with *no gross tumour* at the margins of resection (with or without microscopic involvement)

pT4
Microscopic confirmation of tumour in the pancreas more than 2 cm from the ampulla or invasion of other adjacent organs

Pancreas **pT2 or less**
Pathological examination of the primary carcinoma with *no gross tumour* at the margins of resection (with or without microscopic involvement)

pT3
Microscopic confirmation of invasion of any of the following adjacent tissues: duodenum, bile duct, splenic vessels, peripancreatic tissues

pT4
Microscopic confirmation of invasion of stomach, spleen, colon and/or adjacent large vessels

pN–Regional Lymph Nodes

The site-specific recommendations regarding number of nodes for diagnosis of pN0 for all sites of Digestive System Tumours have been incorporated in the 5th edition [13] (see Table 3).

Site **Recommendations**

Oesophagus **pN1**
Microscopic confirmation of at least one regional lymph node metastasis

Stomach **pN1**
Microscopic confirmation of one to six regional lymph node metastasis

pN2
Microscopic confirmation of seven to fifteen regional lymph node metastasis

pN3
Microscopic confirmation of more than fifteen regional lymph node metastasis

Small intestine

pN1
Microscopic confirmation of at least one regional lymph node metastasis

Colon and rectum

pN1
Microscopic confirmation of one to three regional lymph node metastasis

pN2
Microscopic confirmation of more than three regional lymph node metastasis

pN1/2
If the pathology report does not indicate the number of involved nodes, classify pN1

Anal Canal

pN1
Microscopic confirmation of metastasis in perirectal lymph node(s)

pN2
Microscopic confirmation of metastasis in unilateral internal iliac and/or inguinal lymph node(s)

pN3
Microscopic confirmation of metastasis in perirectal and/or inguinal lymph nodes and/or bilateral internal iliac lymph nodes and/or bilateral inguinal lymph nodes

Liver

pN1
Microscopic confirmation of at least one regional lymph node metastasis

Gallbladder, Extrahepatic Bile Ducts

pN1
Microscopic confirmation of metastasis in lymph node(s) of the hepatoduodenal ligament (cystic duct, pericholedochal, hilar lymph nodes)

pN2
Microscopic confirmation of metastasis in peripancreatic (head only), periduodenal, periportal, coeliac and/or superior mesenteric lymph node(s)

Ampulla of Vater, Pancreas

pN1
Microscopic confirmation of at least one regional lymph node metastasis

Lung and Pleural Tumours

pT–Primary Tumour

Site	Recommendations
Lung Tumours	**pT3 or less** Pathological examination of the primary carcinoma with *no gross tumour* at the margins of resection (with or without microscopic involvement)
	pT4 Microscopic confirmation of invasion of any of the following: mediastinum, heart, great vessels, trachea, oesophagus, vertebral body, carina *or* microscopic confirmation of separate tumour nodule(s) in the same lobe or malignant cells in pleural effusion confirmed by cytology
Pleural Mesothelioma	**pT3 or less** Pathological examination of the primary carcinoma with *no gross tumour* at the margins of resection (with or without microscopic involvement)
	pT4 Microscopic confirmation of invasion of any of the following: contralateral pleura, contralateral lung, peritoneum, intra-abdominal organs, cervical tissues

pN–Regional Lymph Nodes

The site-specific recommendations regarding number of nodes for diagnosis of pN0 for lung tumours have been incorporated in the 5th edition [13] (see Table 3).

Site	Recommendations
Lung Tumours and Pleural Mesothelioma	**pN1** Microscopic confirmation of metastasis in ipsilateral peribronchial lymph node(s) or ipsilateral hilar lymph node(s) [including intrapulmonary lymph nodes for lung]

pN2
Microscopic confirmation of metastasis in ipsilateral mediastinal lymph node(s) or subcarinal lymph node(s)

pN3
Microscopic confirmation of metastasis in contralateral mediastinal lymph node(s) or contralateral hilar lymph node(s) or scalene or supraclavicular lymph node(s) (ipsilateral or contralateral)

Tumours of Bone and Soft Tissues

pT–Primary Tumour

Site	Recommendations
Bone	**pT1** Pathological examination of the primary tumour with *no gross tumour* at the margins of resection (with or without microscopic involvement) **pT2** Microscopic confirmation of invasion beyond the cortex
Soft Tissues	**pT1 and pT2** Pathological examination of the primary tumour with *no gross tumour* at the margins of resection (with or without microscopic involvement)

pN–Regional Lymph Nodes

Site	Recommendations
Bone and Soft Tissues	**pN0** Histological examination of a regional lymphadenectomy specimen which will ordinarily include six or more lymph nodes

pN1
Microscopic confirmation of at least one régional lymph node metastasis

Skin Tumours

pT–Primary Tumour

Tumour type	Recommendations
Carcinoma	**pT3 or less** Pathological examination of the primary carcinoma with *no gross tumour* at the margins of resection (with or without microscopic involvement) **pT4** Microscopic confirmation of invasion of deep extra-dermal structures, i.e., cartilage, skeletal muscle or bone
Malignant Melanoma	**pT3 or less** Pathological examination of the primary melanoma with *no gross tumour* at the lateral margins of resection and with no histological tumour at the deep margins of resection **pT4** Pathological examination of the primary melanoma incompletely removed but more than 4 mm in thickness and/or with invasion of the subcutaneous tissue *or* Microscopic confirmation of satellites (pT4b)

pN–Regional Lymph Nodes

The site-specific recommendations regarding number of nodes for diagnosis of pN0 for all sites of skin tumours have been incorporated in the 5th edition (see Table 3).

Tumour type	Recommendations
Carcinoma	**pN1** Microscopic confirmation of at least one regional lymph node metastasis

Malignant Melanoma   **pN1**
Histological examination of or positive biopsy from a regional lymph node metastasis 3 cm or less in greatest dimension[1]

pN2a
Histological examination of or positive biopsy from a regional lymph node metastasis more than 3 cm in greatest dimension

pN2b
Microscopic confirmation of an in-transit metastasis

pN2c
Metastasis more than 3 cm in greatest dimension in any regional lymph node(s) and microscopic confirmation of in-transit metastasis

[1]**Note.** If the size of the biopsied lymph node(s) is not indicated by the submitting surgeon, classify a positive biopsy from a lymph node as pN1.

Breast Tumours

pT – Primary Tumour

Tumour type	Recommendations
All pT	Pathological examination of the primary carcinoma with no *gross tumour* at the margins of resection (with or without microscopic involvement)

pN – Regional Lymph Nodes

Recommendations:

The site-specific recommendations regarding number of nodes for diagnosis of pN0 for Breast tumours have been incorporated in the 5th edition of TNM [13] (see Table 3).

pN1

Histological examination of at least the low axillary lymph nodes (level I), which will ordinarily include six or more lymph nodes

pN2

Microscopic confirmation of a metastasis to ipsilateral axillary lymph nodes fixed to one another or to other structures

pN3

Microscopic confirmation of a metastasis to ipsilateral internal mammary lymph node(s)

Note. Based on the results of histological examination of 1446 patients with complete axillary dissection [10], a mathematical model was developed by Kiricuta and Tausch [5] to determine the sample size from level I necessary for 90% certainty of N0 axillary status. According to this model the examination of 10 lymph nodes from level I is needed.

Gynaecological Tumours

pT–Primary Tumours

Site	Recommendations
Vulva	**pT3 or less** Pathological examination of the primary carcinoma with *no gross tumour* at the margins of resection (with or without microscopic involvement) **pT4** Microscopic confirmation of invasion of any of the following: bladder mucosa, rectal mucosa, upper-urethral mucosa, pelvic bone
Vagina	**pT3 or less** Pathological examination of the primary carcinoma with *no gross tumour* at the margins of resection (with or without microscopic involvement) **pT4** Microscopic confirmation of invasion of the mucosa of bladder or rectum or of extension beyond the true pelvis
Cervix Uteri and Corpus Uteri	**pT3 or less** Pathological examination of the primary carcinoma with *no gross tumour* at the margins of resection (with or without microscopic involvement) **pT4** Microscopic confirmation of invasion of mucosa of bladder or bowel or (for cervix uteri) beyond the true pelvis

Ovary	**pT1** Pathological examination of both ovaries
	pT2 Microscopic confirmation of tumour outside the ovary within the pelvis or cytologically proven malignant cells in ascites or peritoneal washing
	pT3 Microscopic confirmation of peritoneal metastasis outside the pelvis
Fallopian Tube	**pT1** Pathological examination of both tubes
	pT2 Microscopic confirmation of tumour outside the tube within the pelvis or cytologically proven malignant cells in ascites or peritoneal washing
	pT3 Microscopic confirmation of peritoncal metastasis outside the pelvis

Note. (Ovary and Fallopian tube). In the case of histologically proven tumour on pelvic peritoncum only but macroscopic finding of peritoneal metastasis outside the pelvis by the surgeon, the tumour is classified (c)T3 pT2

pN–Regional Lymph Nodes

The site-specific recommendations regarding number of nodes for diagnosis of pN0 for all gynaecological tumours have been incorporated in the 5th edition [13] (see Table 3).

Site	Recommendations
Vulva	**pN1** Microscopic confirmation of a unilateral regional lymph node metastasis
	pN2 Microscopic confirmation of bilateral regional lymph node metastasis
Vagina, Cervix Uteri, Corpus Uteri, Ovary, Fallopian tube	**pN1** Microscopic confirmation of at least one regional lymph node metastasis

Urological Tumours

pT–Primary Tumour

Site	Recommendations
Penis	**pT3 or less** Pathological examination of the primary carcinoma removed by partial or total penis amputation with *no gross tumour* at the margins of resection (with or without microscopic involvement) *or* Pathological examination of the primary tumour removed by local excision with histologically tumour-free margins of resection **pT4** Microscopic confirmation of invasion of adjacent structures other than urethra or prostate
Prostate	**pT1** A pT1 category is not defined, because there is insufficient tissue to assess the highest T category **pT2 or pT3** Pathological examination of a radical prostatectomy specimen with *no gross tumour* at the margins of resection (with or without microscopic involvement) *or* Pathological examination of a simple prostatectomy specimen with histologically tumour-free margins of resection **pT4** Microscopic confirmation of invasion of adjacent structures other than seminal vesicles: bladder neck, external sphincter, rectum, levator muscles, and/or pelvic wall
Testis	**All pT** Pathological examination of a radical orchiectomy specimen.
Kidney	**pT3 or less** Pathological examination of a partial or total nephrectomy specimen with *no gross tumour* at the margins of resection (with or without microscopic involvement) **pT4** Microscopic confirmation of invasion beyond Gerota fascia

Renal Pelvis and Ureter	**pT3 or less** Pathological examination of the primary carcinoma with *no gross tumour* at the margins of resection (with or without microscopic involvement) **pT4** Microscopic confirmation of invasion of perinephric fat or adjacent organs
Urinary Bladder	**pT3 or less** Pathological examination of partial or total cystectomy specimen with *no gross tumour* at the margins of resection (with or without microscopic involvement) **pT4** Microscopic confirmation of invasion of any of the following: prostate, uterus, vagina, pelvic wall, abdominal wall, intestine, seminal vesicles, or microscopic confirmation of perforation of visceral peritoneum

Note. There is a problem in the classification of bladder tumours after transurethral resection. The precondition for pT can only be met in cases of complete tumour resection, i.e., resection of all grossly visible tumour tissue from the remaining grossly tumour-free adjacent bladder wall (deep and laterally). If these additionally and separately submitted tissues are histologically negative, a complete tumour resection can be assumed. Only in such patients can pTaNXMX, pTisNXMX, pT1MXM0, pT2aNXM0 be considered as pathologic stages.

Urethra	**pT3 or less** Pathological examination of the primary carcinoma with *no gross tumour* at the margins of resection (with or without microscopic involvement) **pT4** Microscopic confirmation of invasion of adjacent organs other than prostate, anterior vagina and bladder neck

pN–Regional Lymph Nodes

The definitions of the following N categories for urological tumours changed between the 4th [12] and 5th [13] editions of TNM.

Site	N Categories (except NX and N0)
Penis	N1, N2, N3
Prostate	N1
Testis	N1, N2, N3, pN1, pN2, pN3
Kidney	N1, N2

Renal pelvis and ureter	N1, N2, N3
Urinary bladder	N1, N2, N3
Urethra	N1, N2

Site	Recommendations
All sites except penis	**pN0** Histological examination of a regional lymphadenectomy specimen which will ordinarily include eight or more lymph nodes (see Table 3).*

Note. Measurements are made of the metastasis, not of the entire lymph node. If the size of *biopsied* lymph node(s) is not indicated by the submitting surgeon, classify as pN1 if there is a positive biopsy from one lymph node and as pN2 (except prostate) if there are positive biopsies from two or more lymph nodes.

Penis	**pN0** Histological examination of an inguinal lymphadenectomy specimen which will ordinarily include six or more lymph nodes **pN1** Microscopic confirmation of metastasis in a single superficial inguinal lymph node **pN2** Microscopic confirmation of metastasis in multiple or bilateral superficial inguinal lymph nodes **pN3** Microscopic confirmation of metastasis in deep inguinal or pelvic lymph node(s)
Prostate	**pN1** Microscopic confirmation of at least one regional lymph node metastasis
Testis	**pN1** Microscopic confirmation of a lymph node metastasis (lymph node mass) 2 cm or less in greatest dimension or at least one/not more than 5 positive lymph nodes, none more than 2 cm in greatest dimension

---

* These recommendations are not included in the 5th TNM edition but are new.

pN2
Microscopic confirmation of a lymph node metastasis (lymph node mass) more than 2 cm in greatest dimension but not more than 5 cm in greatest dimension; or more than 5 nodes positive, none more than 5 cm; or evidence of extranodal extension of tumour

pN3
Microscopic confirmation of a lymph node metastasis (lymph node mass) more than 5 cm in greatest dimension

Kidney

pN1
Microscopic confirmation of a single regional lymph node metastasis

pN2
Microscopic confirmation of metastasis in more than one regional lymph node

Renal pelvis, Ureter, Urinary bladder

pN1
Microscopic confirmation of a single lymph node metastasis not more than 2 cm in diameter

pN2
Microscopic confirmation of a single lymph node metastasis more than 2 cm but not more than 5 cm in greatest dimension *or* Microscopic confirmation of at least two lymph node metastasis, none more than 5 cm in greatest dimension

pN3
Microscopic confirmation of a lymph node metastasis more than 5 cm in greatest dimension

Urethra

pN1
Microscopic confirmation of a single lymph node metastasis 2 cm or less in greatest dimension

pN2
Microscopic confirmation of a single lymph node metastasis more than 2 cm in greatest dimension, *or* Microscopic confirmation of multiple lymph node metastasis

Ophthalmic Tumours

pT–Primary Tumour

Site/Type	Recommendations
Carcinoma of Eyelid	**pT3 or less** Pathological examination of the primary carcinoma with histologically tumour-free margins of resection **pT4** Microscopic confirmation of invasion of adjacent structures
Carcinoma of Conjunctiva	**pT 3 or less** Pathological examination of the primary carcinoma with histologically tumour-free margins of resection **pT4** Microscopic confirmation of invasion of the orbit
Malignant Melanoma of Conjunctiva	**pT3 or less** Pathological examination of the primary melanoma with histologically tumour-free margins of resection **pT4** Microscopic confirmation of invasion of the eyelid, cornea and/or orbit
Malignant Melanoma of Uvea	**pT3 or less** Pathological examination of the primary melanoma with histologically tumour-free margins of resection **pT4** Microscopic confirmation of extraocular extension
Retinoblastoma	**pT3 or less** Pathological examination of the primary retinoblastoma with histologically tumour-free margins of resection **pT4** Microscopic confirmation of intraneural tumour beyond lamina cribrosa but not at the line of resection (pT4a)

	Microscopic confirmation of tumour at the line of resection or other extraocular extension (pT4b)
Sarcoma of Orbit	**pT3 or less** Pathological examination of the primary sarcoma with histologically tumour-free margins of resection
	pT4 Microscopic confirmation of tumour beyond the orbit (adjacent sinuses and/or cranium)
Carcinoma of Lacrimal Gland	**pT3 or less** Pathological examination of the primary carcinoma with *no gross tumour* at the margins of resection (with or without microscopic involvement)
	pT4 Microscopic confirmation of invasion of orbital tissues, optic nerve, or globe, without (pT4a) or with (pT4b) bone invasion

pN–Regional Lymph Nodes

Site	Recommendations
All Sites and Types	**pN0** Histological examination of a regional lymphadenectomy specimen which will ordinarily include six or more lymph nodes
	pN1 Microscopic confirmation of atleast one regional lymph node metastasis

Hodgkin Disease and Non-Hodgkin Lymphomas

Pathological staging requires the histological examination of:

- Liver biopsies
- At least four abdominal lymph nodes
- Bone marrow biopsies from clinically or radiologically non-involved area of bone
- Spleen or spleen biopsies

References

[1] Fielding LP, Arsenault PA, Chapuis PH, et al. Clinicopathological staging for colorectal cancer: an International Documentation System (IDS) and an International Comprehensive Anatomical Terminology (ICAT). *J Gastroenterol Hepatol* 1991; **6**: 325–344

[2] Hermanek P, Giedl J, Dworak O. Two programmes for examination of regional lymph nodes in colorectal carcinoma with regard to the new pN classification. *Pathol Res Pract* 1989; **185**: 867–873

[3] Hermanek P. Onkologische Chirurgie/Pathologisch-anatomische Sicht. *Langenbecks Arch Chir Suppl* 1991; 277–281

[4] Honthoff MJ. Surgical pathology of hepatobiliary and pancreatic tumours. In *Hepatobiliary and Pancreatic Malignancies*, Lygidakis NJ, Tytgat GNJ (eds). Thieme: Stuttgart, 1989

[5] Kiricuta CI, Tausch J. A mathematical model of axillary lymph node involvement based on 1446 complete axillary dissections in patients with breast carcinoma. *Cancer* 1992; **69**: 2496–2501

[6] Qizilbash AH. Pathologic studies in colorectal cancer. *Pathol Annu* 1982; **17**: 1–46

[7] Remmele W. Staging, typing and grading of colorectal cancer: a critical review of current classification systems. *Prog Surg Pathol* 1984; **5**: 7–36

[8] Robbins KT, Medina JE, Wolfe GT, Levine PA, Sessions RB, Pruet CW. Standardizing neck dissection terminology. Official report of the Academy's Committee for Head and Neck Surgery and Oncology. *Arch Otolaryngol Head Neck Surg* 1991; **117**: 601–605

[9] Rosai J. *Ackerman's Surgical Pathology* (8th ed). Mosby: St. Louis, MO, 1996

[10] Veronesi U, Luini A, Galimberti V, Marchini S, Sacchini V, Rilke F. Extent of metastatic axillary involvement in 1446 cases of breast cancer. *Eur J Surg Oncol* 1990; **16**: 127–133

[11] *UICC: TNM Supplement 1993. A commentary on uniform use*. Hermanek P, Henson DE, Hutter RVP, Sobin LH (eds) Springer: Berlin Heidelberg New York Tokyo, 1993

[12] *UICC. TNM Classification of Malignant Tumours*. Hermanek P, Sobin LH (eds) Springer: Berlin Heidelberg New York, 1987, 2nd revision, 1992

[13] *UICC. TNM Classification of Malignant Tumours*. Sobin LH, Wittekind Ch (eds) Wiley-Liss: New York, 1997

[14] Zeng Z, Cohen AM, Hajdu S, et al. Serosal cytologic study to determine free mesothelial penetration by intraperitoneal colon cancer. *Cancer* 1992; **70**: 737–740

New TNM Classifications Recommended for Testing

Introduction

This chapter contains proposals for new classifications as follows:

General

- Perineural invasion

Specific

- Gastrointestinal sarcomas
- Malignant thymoma
- Cranial and facial bones
- Cutaneous T-cell lymphoma
- Chronic myeloid leukaemia
- Primary liver carcinoma in infants and children
- Adrenal cortical carcinoma
- Liver metastasis of colorectal carcinoma
- Gastrointestinal malignant lymphomas

These new classifications are provisional. Testing by several institutions and on large numbers of patients is needed before general acceptance can be recommended. Those having relevant data, published or not, on these classifications are invited to contact the TNM Prognostic Factors Project Committee of the UICC.

General

Perineural Invasion

In a variety of tumours, perineural invasion can be observed and may influence prognosis. This finding has not been separately classified in TNM. As an optional descriptor, a Pn classification is recommended for testing.

Pn Perineural Invasion

PnX   Perineural invasion cannot be assessed
Pn0   No perineural invasion
Pn1   Perineural invasion

Specific

Gastrointestinal Sarcomas (ICD-0 C15-C21)

The classification is based on preliminary data from the SEER Program [15] suggesting the use of the TNM 4th edition classification of soft tissue sarcomas [19, 22] for visceral sarcomas.

Rules for Classification

The classification applies to sarcomas of gastrointestinal hollow viscera. Kaposi sarcoma is not included. There should be histological confirmation of the disease and division of cases by histological type and grade.

The following are the procedures for assessing the T, N and M categories:

T categories   Physical examination, imaging, endoscopy, and/or surgical exploration
N categories   Physical examination, imaging, and/or surgical exploration
M categories   Physical examination, imaging, and/or surgical exploration

Anatomical Sites

1. Oesophagus (C15)
2. Stomach (Cl6)
3. Small intestine (C17)
4. Colon (C18)
5. Rectum (including rectosigmoid junction) (C19, C20)
6. Anal canal (C21)

Regional Lymph Nodes

The regional lymph nodes are those appropriate to the site of the primary tumour.

TNM Clinical Classification

T–Primary Tumour

TX   Primary tumour cannot be assessed
T0   No evidence of primary tumour
Tl   Tumour 5 cm or less in greatest dimension
T2   Tumour more than 5 cm in greatest dimension

N–Regional Lymph Nodes

NX   Regional lymph nodes cannot be assessed

N0   No regional lymph node metastasis
N1   Regional lymph node metastasis

M-Distant Metastasis

MX   Distant metastasis cannot be assessed
M0   No distant metastasis
M1   Distant metastasis

pTNM Pathological Classification

The pT, pN and pM categories correspond to the T, N and M categories.

G Histopathological Grading

GX   Grade of differentiation cannot be assessed
G1   Well differentiated/low grade
G2   Moderately differentiated/intermediate grade
G3   Poorly differentiated/high grade
G4   Undifferentiated/high grade

Note. After the histological type has been determined, the tumour should be graded according to accepted criteria, including particularly mitotic activity.

Stage Grouping

Stage IA	G1	T1	N0	M0
Stage IB	G1	T2	N0	M0
Stage IIA	G2	T1	N0	M0
Stage IIB	G2	T2	N0	M0
Stage IIIA	G3,4	T1	N0	M0
Stage IIIB	G3,4	T2	N0	M0
Stage IVA	Any G	Any T	N1	M0
Stage IVB	Any G	Any T	Any N	M1

Summary

Gastrointestinal Sarcomas

T1	≤ 5 cm
T2	>5 cm
N1	Regional
G1	Well differentiated/low grade
G2	Moderately differentiated/intermediate grade
G3	Poorly differentiated/high grade
G4	Undifferentiated/high grade

Malignant Thymoma (ICD-0 C37)

The classification is based on Japanese data published by Yamakawa et al. (1991) [16, 20].

Rules for Classification

The classification applies only to malignant thymic epithelial tumours (WHO 1999) [12]. Thymic carcinoids, germ cell tumours and malignant lymphoma are excluded from this classification. There should be histological confirmation of the disease and division of cases by histological type.

T categories	Physical examination and imaging, endoscopy and/or surgical exploration
N categories	Physical examination and imaging, endoscopy and/or surgical exploration
M categories	Physical examination and imaging and/or surgical exploration

Regional Lymph Nodes

The regional lymph nodes are the intrathoracic, scalene and supraclavicular nodes.

TNM Clinical Classification

T Primary Tumour

TX   Primary tumour cannot be assessed
T0   No evidence of primary tumour
T1   Tumour completely encapsulated
T2   Tumour invades pericapsular connective tissue
T3   Tumour invades into neighbouring structures, such as pericardium, mediastinal pleura, thoracic wall, great vessels and lung
T4   Tumour with pleural or pericardial dissemination

N Regional Lymph Nodes

NX   Regional lymph nodes cannot be assessed
N0   No regional lymph node metastasis
N1   Metastasis in anterior mediastinal lymph nodes
N2   Metastasis in other intrathoracic lymph nodes
N3   Metastasis in scalene and/or supraclavicular lymph nodes

M Distant Metastasis

MX   Distant metastasis cannot be assessed
M0   No distant metastasis
M1   Distant metastasis

pTNM Pathological Classification

The pT, pN and pM categories correspond to the T, N and M categories.

Stage Grouping

Stage I	T1	N0	M0
Stage II	T2	N0	M0
Stage III	T1	N1	M0
	T2	N1	M0
	T3	N0, 1	M0
Stage IV	T4	Any N	M0
	Any T	N2, 3	M0
	Any T	Any N	M1

Summary

Malignant Thymoma

T1	Completely encapsulated
T2	Pericapsular connective tissue
T3	Neighbouring structures, e.g., pericardium, mediastinal pleura, thorax wall, great vessels, lung
T4	Pleural/pericardial dissemination
N1	Anterior mediastinal
N2	Other intrathoracic
N3	Scalene/supraclavicular

Cranial and Facial Bones (ICD-0 C41.0,1)

The classification is based on the results of a field trial carried out by B. Spiessl, Basel, Switzerland, and W. Piotrowski, Mannheim, Germany, on behalf of the DSK-TNM from 1974 to 1988. The study included 351 patients with malignant tumours (see supporting data, p. 102).

Rules for Classification

There should be histological classification of the disease to permit division of cases by histological type, which is needed for the T classification.

The following are the procedures for assessment of the T, N and M categories:

T categories	Physical examination and imaging
N categories	Physical examination and imaging
M categories	Physical examination and imaging

Anatomical Subsites

1. Bones of skull (C41.0): frontal bone, parietal bone, occipital bone, sphenoid bone, temporal bone
2. Bones of face (C41.0): ethmoid bone, inferior nasal concha, lacrimal bone, maxillary bone, nasal bone, palatine bone, vomer, zygomatic bone
3. Mandible (C41.1)

Histological Types of Tumours

The following histological types of malignant tumours are included in the classification, the appropriate ICD-O morphology rubrics being indicated:

1. Osteosarcomas (9180-9195/3)
2. Other sarcomas:
    a) Malignant fibrous tumours
        Fibrosarcoma (8810/3)
        Fibromyxosarcoma (8811/3)
        Fibrous histiocytoma, malignant (8830/3)
    b) Malignant blood vessel tumours
        Hemangiosarcoma (9120/3)
        Hemangioendothelioma, malignant (9130/3)
        Epithelioid hemangioendothelioma, malignant (9133/3)
        Hemangiopericytoma, malignant (9150/3)
    c) Malignant chondromatous tumours
        Chondrosarcoma (9220/3)
        Chondroblastoma, malignant (9230/3)
        Myxoid chondrosarcoma (9231/3)
        Mesenchymal chondrosarcoma (9240/3)
    d) Malignant odontogenic tumours (9270/3-9342/3)
    e) Malignant nerve sheath tumours
        Peripheral nerve sheath tumour, malignant (9540/3)
        Neurilemmoma, malignant (9560/3)

Regional Lymph Nodes

The regional lymph nodes are the preauricular, submandibular and cervical lymph nodes.

TNM Clinical Classification

T–Primary Tumour

TX   Primary tumour cannot be assessed
T0   No evidence of primary tumour

Osteosarcomas

T1   Tumour limited to mandible
        T1a   Tumour confined within the cortex
        T1b   Tumour invades beyond the cortex
T2   Tumour limited to bones of face
        T2a   Well delimited tumour
        T2b   Poorly delimited tumour
T3   Tumour limited to bones of skull
        T3a   Tumour confined within the cortex
        T3b   Tumour invades beyond the cortex
T4   Tumour involves more than one subsite

Other Sarcomas

T1 Tumour 4 cm or less in greatest dimension
    T1a   Well delimited tumour
    T1b   Poorly delimited tumour
T2 Tumour more than 4 cm in greatest dimension
    T2a   Well delimited tumour
    T2b   Poorly delimited tumour

Note. The subdivisions into a and b are optional. Tumours which are partly well delimited and partly poorly delimited are classified as poorly delimited.

N–Regional Lymph Nodes

NX   Regional lymph nodes cannot be assessed
N0   No regional lymph node metastasis
N1   Regional lymph node metastasis

M–Distant Metastasis

MX   Distant metastasis cannot be assessed
M0   No distant metastasis
M1   Distant metastasis

pTNM Pathological Classification

The pT, pN and pM categories correspond to the T, N and M categories.

Stage Grouping

No stage grouping is at present recommended.

Summary

Cranial and Facial Bones		
	Osteosarcomas	
T1		Limited to mandible
T2		Limited to facial bones
T3		Limited to skull
T4		More than one subsite
	Other Sarcomas	
T1		≤4 cm
	T1a	Well delimited
	T1b	Poorly delimited
T2		>4 cm
	T2a	Well delimited
	T2b	Poorly delimited
	All Types	
N1		Regional

Addendum

The results of the German field trial (Spiessl and Piotrowski) may be summarized as follows:

1. According to a multivariate regression analysis histology, tumour site, tumour size and delimitation are independent prognostic factors.
2. The most important prognostic factor in osteosarcoma is tumour site, tumours of the mandible having a better prognosis than those of bones of face and those of skull ($p = 0.024$).
3. In other sarcomas, tumour size is the most important prognostic factor, sarcomas of ≤ 4 cm having a better prognosis than those with >4 cm tumour size ($p = 0.029$).
4. In osteosarcoma and other sarcomas, invasion beyond cortex and poor delimitation of tumour show a trend to worsening of prognosis, but statistical significance was not achieved.

Cutaneous T-Cell Lymphoma (Excluding Lip, Eyelid, Vulva and Penis) (ICD-0 C44.2-8, C63.2)

A TNM classification for mycosis fungoides of the skin was proposed by the American Mycosis Fungoides Study Group in 1979 [1]. It was used for T-cell lymphomas other than mycosis fungoides by the European Organization for Research and Treatment of Cancer/German Federal Ministry for Research and Technology Cutaneous Lymphoma Group [2]. The N classification is not consistent with the principles of the TNM system used for other anatomical sites or entities. Therefore, in the following classification, the N categories differ from those in the classification of the American Mycosis Fungoides Study Group. However, a "translation" is easily possible (see following table), and stage grouping is not influenced:

American Mycosis Fungoides Study Group	Proposed TNM
N0	N0, pN0
N1	N1, pN0
N2	N0, pN1
N3	N1, pN1

Note. The definitions of T and M and stage grouping are identical in both classifications.

Rules for Classification

The classification applies to any type of cutaneous T-cell lymphoma. There should be histological confirmation of the disease.

The following are the procedures for assessment of T, N and M categories:

T categories	Physical examination, mapping of skin lesions and skin biopsies
N categories	Physical examination, imaging and biopsy
M categories	Physical examination, imaging and biopsy (e.g., bone marrow or liver)

Anatomical Sites

The following sites are identified by the ICD-0 topography rubrics:

1. External ear and other parts of face (excluding lip and eyelid) (C44.2, 3)
2. Scalp and neck (C44.4)
3. Trunk (including anal margin and perianal skin) (C44.5)
4. Upper limb and shoulder (C44.6)
5. Lower limb and hip (C44.7)
6. Scrotum (C63.2)

Regional Lymph Nodes

The regional lymph nodes are the superficial nodes, i.e., those of head and neck (preauricular, submandibular, cervical), and the axillary, epitrochlear, inguinal and popliteal nodes.

TNM Clinical Classification

T–Primary Tumour

TX	Primary tumour cannot be assessed
T0	No evidence of primary tumour
T1	Limited plaques, papules, or eczematous patches covering less than 10% of the skin surface
T2	Disseminated plaques, papules or erythematous patches covering 10% or more of the skin surface
T3	Tumour(s) (one or more)
T4	Generalized erythroderma

Note. When characteristics of more than one T category exist, the highest is used for classification.

Definitions (International League of Dermatological Societies 1987 [6])

Plaque	Flat or elevated lesion with increased consistency
Papule	Small, elevated nodular lesion 1 cm or less in greatest dimension
Patch	Change of skin colour larger than "macule" would suggest
Tumour	Nodular lesion more than 1 cm in greatest dimension
Macule	Area of discoloration

Erythroderma   Generalized redness of skin, often combined with scaling and
             edema

N–Regional Lymph Nodes

NX   Regional lymph nodes cannot be assessed
N0   No involvement of regional lymph nodes
N1   Involvement of regional lymph nodes

M–Nonregional Extracutaneous Involvement ("Distant Metastasis")

MX   Nonregional extracutaneous involvement cannot be assessed
M0   No nonregional extracutaneous involvement
M1   Nonregional extracutaneous involvement

pTNM Pathological Classification

The pT, pN and pM categories correspond to the T, N and M categories.

Stage Grouping

Stage IA	T1	N0	pN0, X	M0
Stage IB	T2	N0	pN0, X	M0
Stage IIA	T1	N1	pN0, X	M0
	T2	N1	pN0, X	M0
Stage IIB	T3	Any N	pN0, X	M0
Stage III	T4	Any N	pN0, X	M0
Stage IVA	Any T	Any N	pN1	M0
Stage IVB	Any T	Any N	Any pN	M1

Note. For comparison with the original Classification of the American Mycosis Fungoides Study
Group [1], see Introduction, p. 102.

Summary

Cutaneous T-Cell Lymphoma
T1   Limited plaques, papules or patches (<10% of skin surface)
T2   Disseminated plaques, papules or patches (≥10% of skin surface)
T3   Tumour(s)
T4   Generalized erythroderma
N1   Regional

Chronic Myeloid Leukaemia

The following classification [13] has been recommended for testing by the AJCC
and the UICC. It is based on three parameters, i.e., T (tumour), F (risk factors)
and E (extramedullary tumour). N and M classifications do not apply to this
entity.

Rules for Classification

The classification applies only to chronic myeloid leukaemia. There must be haematological confirmation of the disease.

The following are the procedures for assessing the T, F and E categories:

T categories   Blood and bone marrow examination

F categories   Platelet count, haemoglobin value, basophil count, karyotype or bcr/abl gene rearrangement analysis

E categories   Physical examination, imaging, histology or cytology of extramedullary site(s)

Staging Criteria

T-Tumour

T1	5% or less blasts in bone marrow or blood
T2	More than 5% but not more than 15% blasts in bone marrow or blood
T3	More than 15% but not more than 30% blasts in bone marrow or blood
T4	More than 30% blasts in bone marrow or blood

F-Risk Factors

The risk factors (other than T or E) that may affect outcome are:

- Platelets <100 gpt/l*
- Haemoglobin <7 mg/dl
- Basophilia >20%
- Karyotypic evolution

F0   No risk factor
F1   One risk factor
F2   More than one risk factor

E-Extramedullary Tumour

E0   No extramedullary tumour, or tumour with 30% or fewer blasts in an extramedullary site
E1   Tumour with >30% blasts in an extramedullary site

Stage Grouping

Phase	Stage			
	IA	T1	F0	E0
Chronic	{			
	IB	T2	F0	E0

---

* Platelets gpt/l = gigaparticle/liter, Haemoglobin mg/dl = miligram/deziliter

		T	F	E
Accelerated	IIA	T1	F1	E0
		T1	F2	E0
		T2	F1	E0
	IIB	T2	F2	E0
		T3	Any F	E0
Blastic (acute)	IIIA	T4	Any F	E0
	IIIB	Any T	Any F	El

Summary

Chronic Myeloid Leukaemia

T1	≤5% blasts
T2	>5% to 15% blasts
T3	>15% to 30% blasts
T4	>30% blasts
F0	No risk factor
F1	One risk factor
F2	More than one risk factor
E0	No extramedullary tumour or extramedullary tumour ≤30% blasts
El	Extramedullary tumour >30% blasts

Definitions and Explanatory Notes

Definitions

Chronic myeloid leukaemia (CML) is a haematopoietic malignancy characterized by an increase in peripheral blood cell counts, bone marrow hypercellularity and a *bcr/abl* gene fusion detected either by molecular techniques or by karyotypic analysis for the Philadelphia chromosome. Other myeloproliferative syndromes such as essential thrombocytosis which are positive for *bcr/abl* will be considered as CML. So-called atypical CML and juvenile CML which are negative for *bcr/abl* will be treated as a non-CML myelodysplastic syndrome. Thus CML may be considered as one of the first diseases essentially to be defined by the presence of an acquired gene defect which is best detected by molecular diagnostics. This gene defect, the fusion of the *bcr* gene on chromosome 22 with the *abl* oncogene from chromosome 9, was recognized as an abnormal chromosomal translocation, the Philadelphia chromosome, years before the development of recombinant DNA technology. Research, including transgenic mouse models of CML, has shown that the *bcr/abl* fusion gene produces an abnormal protein which is related to the pathogenesis of the bone marrow neoplastic proliferation.

Clinical

CML may have a prolonged unrecognized preclinical stage. The disease usually presents in a chronic phase (defined in this classification as Stage I) which may be associated with symptoms such as abdominal fullness due to splenomegaly. Alternately, many cases of CML are initially asymptomatic and are detected by a complete blood count performed for unrelated reasons. The chronic phase has a quite variable duration lasting from months to many years with a median duration of 3–4 years. The chronic phase evolves through an accelerated phase (defined as Stage II) characterized by increasing immaturity of the white blood cells in the blood or marrow. Because the accelerated phase is invariable followed by the life-threatening acute phase (defined as Stage III), more drastic therapeutic measures are instituted at this point. Death from CML is usually due to blastic infiltration and haemorrhage or infection in Stage III [17].

Rationale for Staging

The purpose of a staging system is to recognize the life history of a tumour and to apply that knowledge to a particular patient. CML is recognized to have three distinct clinical phases. To study this disease and the effects of new therapies, it is necessary that these phases be accurately described in a staging system. Physicians wishing to provide new therapies for their patients must know how to compare them to the results described in clinical trials. The proposed staging system for monitoring of CML patients defines three stages in a manner which conforms with clinical studies of the progression of this disease. Similar to the standard anatomically based TNM staging of cancer, the CML staging system uses three factors as indices which are then combined into a single stage.

Primary Liver Carcinoma in Infants and Children

The following classification has been proposed by the Japanese TNM Committee. It is based on the examination in 136 cases of hepatoblastoma seen in 14 Japanese institutions [10].

The German Society for Pediatric Oncology and Hematology (GPOH) has recommended use of the TNM classification of primary liver carcinomas for hepatoblastomas [14].

Rules for Classification

The classification applies to primary liver carcinoma in patients age 16 years or younger. In this age, predominantly hepatoblastoma is observed, whereas hepatocellular carcinoma is uncommon. There should be histological verification of the disease.

The following are the procedures for assessment of the T, N and M categories:

T categories   Physical examination, imaging and/or surgical exploration
N categories   Physical examination, imaging and/or surgical exploration
M categories   Physical examination, imaging and/or surgical exploration

Regional Lymph Nodes

The regional lymph nodes are the suprahepatic, infrahepatic, hilar, hepatoduodenal, pancreaticoduodenal and coeliac nodes.

TNM Clinical Classification

T–Primary Tumour

TX   Primary tumour cannot be assessed
T0   No evidence of primary tumour
T1   Tumour confined to one segment of the liver
T2   Tumour confined to two segments of the liver
T3   Tumour confined to three segments of the liver
T4   Tumour involving more than three segments of the liver

Note. For staging purposes the liver is subdivided into 8 segments [3].

N–Regional Lymph Nodes

NX   Regional lymph nodes cannot be assessed
N0   No regional lymph node metastasis
N1   Metastasis to suprahepatic, infrahepatic, hilar or hepatoduodenal lymph nodes
N2   Metastasis to pancreaticoduodenal or coeliac lymph nodes

M–Distant Metastasis

MX   Distant metastasis cannot be assessed
M0   No distant metastasis
M1   Distant metastasis

pTNM Pathological Classification

The pT, pN and pM categories correspond to the T, N and M categories.

Stage Grouping

Stage I	T1	N0	M0
Stage II	T2	N0	M0
Stage IIIA	T3	N0	M0
Stage IIIB	T1	N1,2	M0

	T2	N1,2	M0
	T3	N1,2	M0
	T4	Any N	M0
Stage IV	Any T	Any N	M1

Summary

Primary Liver Carcinoma in Infants and Children	
Tl	1 segment
T2	2 segments
T3	3 segments
T4	>3 segments
Nl	Suprahepatic, infrahepatic, hilar, hepatoduodenal
N2	Pancreaticoduodenal, coeliac

Adrenal Cortical Carcinoma

The classification applies to adrenal cortical carcinoma. This classification is based on data from Henley et al. [4], Sullivan et al. [18], Wooten et al. [23] and Wachenberg et al. [21]. It is also included in the "Recommendations for reporting of tumours of the adrenal cortex and medulla" by the Association of Directors of Anatomy and Surgical Pathology [9].

T–Primary Tumour

TX   Primary tumour cannot be assessed
T0   No evidence of primary tumour
T1   Tumour 5 cm or less, no invasion beyond adrenal
T2   Tumour greater than 5 cm, no invasion beyond adrenal
T3   Tumour of any size, locally invasive but not involving adjacent organs
T4   Tumour of any size, with invasion of adjacent organs

N–Regional Lymph Nodes

NX   Regional lymph nodes cannot be assessed
N0   No regional lymph node metastasis
Nl   Regional lymph node metastasis

M–Distant Metastasis

MX   Distant metastasis cannot be assessed
M0   No distant metastasis
Ml   Distant metastasis

pTNM Pathological Classification

The pT, pN and pM categories correspond to the T, N and M categories.

Stage Grouping

Stage I	Tl	N0	M0
Stage II	T2	N0	M0
Stage III	Tl	N1	M0
	T2	N1	M0
	T3	N0	M0
Stage IV	T4	N0	M0
	T3	N1	M0
	Any T	Any N	M1

Summary

Adrenal Cortical Carcinoma

T1	≤5 cm, no invasion beyond adrenal
T2	>5 cm, no invasion beyond adrenal
T3	Tumour of any size, locally invasive but not involving adjacent organs
T4	Tumour of any size, invasion of adjacent organs
Nl	Regional lymph node metastasis

Liver Metastasis of Colorectal Carcinoma

In a growing number of patients, liver metastasis of colorectal carcinoma can be cured by resective surgery or can be treated palliatively by a variety of treatment methods. Therefore, a more detailed approach for classification than only M1/pM1 is needed. The proposed classification is based on results of a study by Hermanek et al. [5].

Clinical

M2a *Colon tumour*: no regional tumour, only one liver lobe with metastasis, local stage (stage I and II) at primary diagnosis
Rectum tumour: no regional tumour, only one liver lobe with metastasis
M2b Neither M2a nor M2c
M2c Locoregional tumour or metastasis in both lobes or more than five liver metastases

Pathological

pM2a No locoregional tumour, liver metastasis ≤5 cm
pM2b No locoregional tumour, liver metastasis >5 cm *or* locoregional tumour

Gastrointestinal Malignant Lymphomas

This classification is based on the report of a workshop convened to discuss the pathological and staging classifications of gastrointestinal tract malignant lymphoma (Rohatiner et al. [11]). The classification was adopted as proposed by Isaacson [7, 8].

Stage

Stage I   Tumour confined to GI tract
            Single primary site or multiple, noncontiguous lesions in one organ
Stage II   Tumour extending into abdomen from primary GI site
            Nodal involvement
Stage II$_1$ Local (paragastric in cases of gastric lymphoma and paraintestinal for intestinal lymphoma)
Stage II$_2$ Distant (mesenteric in the case of an intestinal primary; otherwise: para-aortic, paracaval, pelvic, inguinal)
Stage II$_E$ Penetration of serosa to involve adjacent organs or tissues (enumerate actual site of involvement, e.g., II$_E$ [pancreas], II$_E$ [large intestine], II$_E$ [post abdominal wall])
Stage IV   Disseminated extranodal involvement, or a GI tract lesion with supradiaphragmatic involvement

Note. Where there is both nodal involvement and penetration to involve adjacent organs, stage should be denoted using both a subscript (1 or 2) and E, e.g., II$_{1E}$ [pancreas].

References

[1] Bunn PA, Lamberg SI. Report of the committee on staging and classification of cutaneous T-cell lymphomas. *Cancer Treatment Rep* 1979; **63**: 725–728

[2] Burg G, Sterry W. EORTC/BMFI Cutaneous Lymphoma Project Group. *Recommendations for staging and therapy of cutaneous lymphomas. A European concept*. EORTC/BMFT, Würzburg, 1987)

[3] Couinaud C. *Le foie. Etudes anatomiques et chirurgicales*. Masson: Paris, 1957

[4] Henley DJ, van Heerden JA, Grant CS, Carney JA, Carpenter PC. Adrenocortical carcinoma — A continuing challenge. *Surgery* 1983; **94**: 926–931

[5] Hermanek P. Liver metastases: Classification and staging systems. *HepatoGastroenterol* 1992; **39**: 10–17

[6] International League of Dermatological Societies, Committee on Nomenclature. *Glossary of basic dermatology lesions*. Almquist and Wiksell: Uppsala, 1987

[7] Isaacson P, Wright DH. Malignant lymphoma of mucosa associated lymphoid tissue. *Cancer* 1983; **53**: 2515–2514

[8] Isaacson P, Spencer G, Wright DH. Classifying primary gut lymphomas. *Lancet* 1988; **12**: 1148–1149

[9] Lack EE, Askin B, Dehner LP, et al. Recommendations for reporting of tumours of the adrenal cortex and medulla. *Hum Pathol* 1999; **30**: 887–890

[10] Morita K, Okabe I, Uchino J, et al. The proposed JapaneseTNM lassification of primary liver carcinoma in infants and children. *Jpn J Clin Oncol* 1983; **13**: 361–370

[11] Rohatiner A, on behalf of d'Amore F, Coiffier B, Crowther D, Gospodarowicz MK, Isaacson P, Lister TA, Norton A, Salem P, Shipp M, Somers R. Report on a workshop convened to discuss the pathological and staging classifications of gastrointestinal tract lymphoma. *Ann Oncol* 1994; **5**: 397–400

[12] Rosai J. Histological typing of tumours of the thymus (2nd ed). *WHO International Histological Typing of Tumours*. Springer: Berlin Heidelberg New York, 1999

[13] Ross DN, Brunning RD, Kantarjian HM, Koeffler HP, Ozer H. A proposed staging system for chronic myeloid leukemia. *Cancer* 1993; **71**: 388–3791

[14] von Schweinitz D, Hecker H, Schmidt-von Arndt G, Harms D. Prognostic factors and staging systems in childhood hepatoblastoma. *Int J Cancer* 1997; **74**: 593–599

[15] *SEER Program: Code manual*. Third edition NIH Publication No 98-2313. National Cancer Institute: Bethesda, 1998

[16] Shimosato Y, Mukai K. Tumours of Mediastinum. 3rd series, Fascicle 21, *Atlas of Tumour Pathology* (1997). AFIP, Washington

[17] Sokal JE, Cox EB, Baccarani M, et al. Prognostic discrimination in "good-risk" chronic granulocytic leukemia. *Blood* 1984; **63**: 789–799

[18] Sullivan M, Boileau M, Hodges CV. Adrenal cortical carcinoma. *J Urol* 1978; **120**: 660–665

[19] *UICC (International Union against Cancer) TNM classification of Malignant Tumours* (4th ed) Hermanek P, Sobin LH (eds). Springer: Berlin Heidelberg New York 1987, 2nd revision 1992

[20] Yamakawa Y, Masaoka A, Hashimoto T, Niwa H, Muzino T, Fujii Y, Nakahara K. A tentative tumour-node-metastasis classification of thymoma. *Cancer* 1991; **68**: 1984–1987

[21] Wachenberg BL, Arbergaria Pereira MA, Modona BB, et al. Adrenocortical carcinoma. Clinical and laboratory observations. *Cancer* 2000; **88**: 711–736

[22] Weiss SW. Histological Typing of Soft Tissue Tumours. In *WHO International Histological Classification of Tumours*. Springer: Berlin Heidelberg New York, 1994

[23] Wooten MD, King DK. Adrenal cortical carcinoma. Epidemiology and treatment with mitotane and a review of the literature. *Cancer* 1993; **72**: 3145–3155

Optional Proposals for Testing New Telescopic Ramifications of TNM

In this chapter, various proposals for optional subdivision of the existing T, N and M categories, i.e., "telescopic" ramification, are presented. Telescoping accommodates the collection of additional data without altering the definitions of the existing TNM categories.

The concept of telescoping permits an orderly expansion of TNM elements to allow for (1) testing of subcategories for prognosis and (2) treatment planning considerations. Telescoping accommodates "splitters" and "lumpers", permits data from expansions to collapse into the standard categories and promotes testing of new hypotheses uniformly in different centres.

The editors recognize that staging must be simple enough for universal use in both highly developed and developing countries and sufficiently uncomplicated so that medical professionals are not discouraged from using the system. On the other hand, for specialized institutions and for investigational purposes a relatively simple staging system is not sufficient and runs the risk of not being used. For these specialized institutions the TNM system may be made more attractive by further subdivision of the existing categories (telescopic ramification) and by including additional descriptors.

The proposals for subdivisions and additional designations in this section are presented for investigational use and are *entirely optional*. Some proposals relate to subclassifications of M1 and are of interest to oncologists. Justification for each proposal is given based on published data or clinical experience.

All Tumour Sites

Fixation of Lymph Nodes

Some clinicians believe that fixation of lymph nodes to adjacent structures is important for treatment planning. For analysis, fixation may be specified within the existing N categories, e.g., N1, N2 or N3.

Micrometastasis

pN1   Cases with micrometastasis only, i.e. no metastasis larger than 0.2 cm, can be identified by the addition of "(mi)", e.g., pNl(mi) or pN2(mi).

In breast cancer this does not apply because size of metastasis is already considered in the pN classification.

pM1   Micrometastasis, i.e., no metastasis larger than 0.2 cm, in viscera (lung, liver, etc.) or bone marrow can be identified by the addition of "(mi)", e.g., pM1(mi).

Justification. Historical considerations, general experience.

For the distinction between micrometastasis and isolated tumour cells see Hermanek et al 1999 [19]. For recording the presence of isolated tumour cells see p. 7.

Markers of Residual Tumour

R0   R0a   Negative markers after tumour resection for cure (R0)
R0b   Persistently elevated marker level or rising marker level within 4 months after tumour resection for cure

Justification. General considerations, general experience (DSK-TNM).

Head and Neck Tumours

Thyroid Gland

T Classification

Tl,2,3a,b   (i)   Grossly encapsulated tumour
(ii)   Grossly nonencapsulated tumour

Justification. Different prognosis and treatment, especially for follicular carcinoma in patients under 45 years (ECC).

N Classification

Nla   (i)   Metastasis in ipsilateral central cervical lymph nodes
(ii)   Metastasis in ipsilateral lateral cervical lymph nodes

Note. The *central* cervical lymph nodes are the submandibular, submental, prelaryngeal and paratracheal (supra-, peri-, infrathyroidal, pretracheal) lymph nodes. The *lateral* cervical lymph nodes are the superficial and deep lateral cervical and the supraclavicular nodes.

Justification. Treatment planning (Dralle et al. 1994 [7]).

Digestive System Tumours

All Sites Except Oesophagus, Colon and Rectum

M Classification

M1   M1a   Metastasis in non-regional lymph nodes only
     M1b   Metastasis in viscera (excluding peritoneal and pleural
           metastasis)
     M1c   Peritoneal or pleural metastasis

Justification. Different prognosis, response to chemotherapy, and treatment
(ECC).

Oesophagus

T Classification

T1   T1a   Tumour invades lamina propria
     T1b   Tumour invades submucosa

Justification. Different frequency of lymph node metastasis, different prognosis,
important indication for treatment by laser and limited endoscopic procedures
(Endo et al. [9], Hirayama and Mori [21]; Yoshinaka et al. [46], Torres et al.
[45])

N Classification

N1   N1a   1–3 nodes involved
     N1b   4–7 nodes involved
     N1c   >7 nodes involved

Justification. Different prognosis in relation to the number of involved lymph
nodes demonstrated by Siewert 1992: Squamous cell carcinoma of the intrathoracic oesophagus treated by surgical resection (any R), surgical mortality not
excluded (Kaplan-Meier):

	Number of patients	2-year survival rate (%)	5-year survival rate (%)	Median survival time (months)
pN1a	58	22	11	12
pN1b	32	18	0	9
pN1c	19	0	0	6

The difference was statistically significant (p <0.05).
    The importance of the number of involved lymph nodes has been confirmed
by Kato et al. [26], and Roder et al. [39].

Stomach

T Classification

T1   T1a   Tumour invades lamina propria (mucosa)
      T1b   Tumour invades submucosa

Justification. ECC: different frequency of lymph node metastasis, different treatment, important as indication for treatment by limited procedures (Inoue et al.) [25].

T2   T2a   Tumour invades muscularis propria
      T2b   Tumour invades subserosa

Justification. ECC: Stomach carcinoma, any type, treated by resection for cure (R0), survival observed, surgical mortality not excluded (Kaplan-Meier):

	Number of patients	*2-year survival rate ± standard error (%)*	*5-year survival rate ± standard error (%)*	*Median survival time (months)*
pT2a	84	74 ± 5	62 ± 6	118.6
pT2b	306	57 ± 3	40 ± 4	36.4

The difference was statistically significant ($p < 0.01$).

Siewert et al [43] reported similar survival rates as from the Erlangen Cancer Center (ECC) with a 5-year survival rate of 62% for pT2a tumours and 41% for pT2b tumours. Harrison et al. [15] reported better prognosis for gastric adenocarcinoma limited to the muscularis propria and confirmed this finding by multivariate analysis.

N Classification

The N Classification, in the TNM 5th edition, is based on number of nodes involved. Some Japanese researchers have proposed the following ramification of the present N categories according to the site of the involved nodes

N1   1 to 6 nodes involved
      N1a   Lymph node metastasis in lymph node positions 1 to 6 only
      N1b   Lymph node metastasis in lymph node positions 7 to 12, too
N2   7 to 15 nodes involved
      N2a   Lymph node metastasis in lymph node positions 1 to 6 only
      N2b   Lymph node metastasis in lymph node positions 7 to 12, too
N3   more than 15 lymph nodes involved
      N3a   Lymph node metastasis in lymph node positions 1 to 6 only
      N3b   Lymph node metastasis in lymph node positions 7 to 12, too

See definition of lymph node groups according to JGCA, Chapter 2, p. 35.

Justification. The purpose of this classification is to enable comparisons between data based on classification of the Japanese Gastric Cancer Association and data based on the TNM classification.

Most authors emphasize simplicity, reduction of methodic problems, less subjectivity and thus, higher reproducibility of the 1997 stomach tumour N classification [20]. The proposal above should provide evidence as to whether the ramification of N categories according to the anatomical position of lymph nodes adds further information to the N categories.

Colon and Rectum

pT Classification

	pT1a	Lymph vessel/blood vessel invasion absent*
	pT1b	Lymph vessel/blood vessel invasion present
pT3	pT3a Minimal:	Tumour invades through the muscularis propria into the subserosa or into nonperitonealized pericolic or perirectal tissues, not more than 1 mm beyond the outer border of muscularis propria
	pT3b Slight.	Tumour invades through the muscularis propria into the subserosa or into nonperitonealized pericolic or perirectal tissues, more than 1 mm but not more than 5 mm beyond the outer border of muscularis propria
	pT3c Moderate:	Tumour invades through the muscularis propria into the subserosa or into nonperitonealized pericolic or perirectal tissues, more than 5 mm but not more than 15 mm beyond the outer border of the muscularis propria
	pT3d Extensive:	Tumour invades through the muscularis propria into the subserosa or into nonperitonealized pericolic or perirectal tissues, more than 15 mm beyond outer border of muscularis propria

Justification. The extent of perimuscular invasion seems to influence prognosis, especially in rectum carcinoma, but such reports are still controversial (Fielding et al. [10]). Therefore, further studies are needed. Krook et al. [29] subdivided pT3 into microscopic and gross involvement and adherence to adjacent organs.

Cawthorn et al. 1990 [6] reported the following 5-year survival for resected rectum carcinoma patients (any R):

---

* Yarbro JW, Page DL, Fielding LP et al. American Joint Committee on Cancer Prognostic Factors Consensus Conference. Cancer 1999; 86: 2436–2446

Invasion beyond muscularis propria	Stage II (pN0)	Stage III (pN1-3)	Total
≤ 4 mm	66%	30%	55%
>4 mm	37%	18%	25%

In the ERCRC and SGCRC studies the perimuscular invasion was subdivided according to histological measurements into ≤ 5, >5 to 15 and >15 mm, in the Swiss Registration Study Colorectal Cancer (SAKK study) into ≤ 5 and >5 mm. The respective unpublished data are as follows:

- SAKK: colon and rectum carcinoma, pN0 only, observed survival 30 months (Kaplan-Meier, surgical mortality not excluded):

  ≤ 5 mm (n = 143)90%;
  >5 mm (n = 106) 62%

- ERCRC, 1978-1988, radical resection for cure (R0), 5-year survival rates (Kaplan-Meier, surgical mortality not excluded):

Tumour site, pN	Extension of perimuscular invasion (mm)	Number of patients	5-year survival rate standard error (%)		
			Observed	Relative	
Rectum	≤ 5	134	75.5 ± 4.8	92 ± 5.8	$p<0.01$
pN0	>5	133	62.2 ± 4.9	75.7 ± 5.9	
Rectum	≤ 5	102	52.8 ± 6.4	63.6 ± 7.7	$p<0.01$
pN 1-3	>5	212	37.2 ± 4.2	44.3 ± 4.9	
Colon	≤ 5	106	89.3 ± 4.1	100 ± 3.7	n. s.
pN0	>5	163	83.1 ± 3.6	100 ± 2.5	
Colon	≤ 5	35	53.3 ± 12.5	62.4 ± 13.5	n. s
pN 1-3	>5	179	54.3 ± 4.7	67.2 ± 5.8	

- SGCRC; 1984-1986, radical resection for cure (R0), 5-year survival rates (Kaplan-Meier, surgical mortality not excluded):

Tumour site, pN	Extension of perimuscular invasion (mm)	Number of patients	5-year survival rate standard error (%)		
			Observed	Relative	
Rectum	≤ 5	128	58.9 ± 4.8	75.0 ± 6.1	n. s.
pN0	>5	115	58.6 ± 5.1	72.1 ± 6.2	
Rectum	≤ 5	76	47.0 ± 6.0	59.7 ± 7.6	$p<0.05$
pN1-3	>5	183	31.9 ± 3.6	38.6 ± 4.3	
Colon	≤ 5	112	70.5 ± 4.7	92.2 ± 6.1	n. s.
pN0	>5	232	66.3 ± 3.4	89.2 ± 4.6	
Colon	≤ 5	42	52.4 ± 7.9	65.3 ± 9.9	n. s.
pN1-3	>5	201	42.4 ± 3.8	56.2 ± 5.0	

For further investigation, a subdivision into 4 subgroups is recommended because of general considerations, although supporting data are not available. For those preferring a simpler subdivision, pT3a and b as well as pT3c and d may be combined.

pT4 pT4a Invasion of adjacent organs or structures, without perforation of visceral peritoneum

  pT4b Perforation of visceral peritoneum

Justification. Unpublished data of the ERCRC showed the following frequencies of distant metastasis: pT4 a, 66/211 (31.3%); pT4b, 107/208 (51.4%). The prognosis following resection for cure (R0), surgical mortality not excluded, was as follows (Kaplan-Meier).

	Number of patients	5-year survival rate standard error (%)		Median survival time (months)
		Observed	*Relative*	
pT4aM0	83	49 ± 7	60 ± 9	58.2
pT4bM0	93	43 ± 8	53 ± 9	46.2
pT4aM1	13	12 ± 11	14 ± 13	22.7
pT4bM1	24	0	0	15.5

The differences were not statistically significant.

Unpublished data from the Concord Hospital, Sydney, Australia, showed a significant influence in multivariate analyses (Chapuis 1992).

Liver

T Classification

T4

  T4a Multiple tumours in more than one lobe, none more than 2 cm in greatest dimension

  T4b Multiple tumours in more than one lobe, any more than 2 cm in greatest dimension

  T4c Tumour(s) involving a major branch of the portal or hepatic vein(s)

  T4d Tumour(s) involving adjacent organ(s) (excluding gallbladder)

  T4e Tumour with perforation of visceral peritoneum

  T4f More than one subcategory

Justification. Japanese report at the UICC TNM Meeting 1989, DSK-TNM.

There are several proposals to change the existing TNM classification particularly with respect to stage grouping.

A proposal of Marsh et al. [31] modified the existing stage grouping

Stage	Vascular invasion	Lobar involvement	Tumour size	Lymph node status	Distant Metastasis
I	None	One lobe	Any	N0	M0
I	None	Two lobes	≤ 2 cm	N0	M0
I	Micro.	One/two lobes	≤ 2 cm	N0	M0
II	Micro.	One lobe	>2 cm	N0	M0
IIIA	None	Two lobes	>2 cm	N0	M0
IIIB	Micro.	Two lobes	>2 cm	N0	M0
IVA	Macro.	One/two lobes	Any	N0	M0
IVB	Micro./Macro.	One/two lobes	Any	N1	M1
IVB	–	–	–	N1	M0
IVB	–	–	–	N0	M1

Micro. = Microscopically, Macro. = Macroscopically

Survival-dependent stage grouping according to the Marsh et al. proposal [31]

Stage	Tumour free survival time (months)
I	190,9
II	127,7
IIIA	69,1
IIIB	37,5
IVA	16,4
IVB	5,3

In accordance with the proposal of Marsh et al. [31], Nozaki et al. [36] also recommended placing positive lymph nodes in stage group IV for intrahepatic cholangiocarcinoma.

Extrahepatic Bile Ducts

T Classification

T3

T3a   Tumour invades gallbladder (no other adjacent structures)

T3b   Tumour invades adjacent structures other than gallbladder (liver, pancreas, duodenum, colon, stomach)

Justification. Different treatment, different prognosis (ECC).

Lung Tumours

M Classification

M1   M1a   Separate tumour nodule(s) in a different lobe (ipsilateral or contralateral)

M1b   Other distant metastasis

Justification. For treatment planning, different prognosis, according to data of Bülzebruck et al. 1999 [5].

Tumours of Bone and Soft Tissues

Bone

T Classification

T1,T2   a   Tumour 15 cm or less in greatest dimension

b   Tumour more than 15 cm in greatest dimension

Justification. Different prognosis according to JJC report 1992 (unpublished data of H. Fukuma).

T2   (i)   Beyond cortex to periosteum

(ii)   Beyond periosteum to surrounding soft tissues

(iii)   With extension to major vessels or nerves

Justification. ICC report 1989, for treatment planning.

Skin Tumours

Carcinoma of Skin

T Classification

T1–3   a   Limited to dermis and 2 mm or less in thickness

b   Limited to dermis and more than 2 mm but not more than 6 mm in thickness

c   Invading the subcutis and/or more than 6 mm in thickness

T4   a   6 mm or less in thickness

b   More than 6 mm in thickness

Justification. This subdivision seems important for treatment planning as it correlates with the risk of regional lymph node metastasis (Breuninger et al.) [3, 4].

Category   Frequency of regional lymph node metastasis during
              follow-up of 2-13 years (median 6.5 years)

T1a	0
T1b	4.5%
T1c	15-20%
T3c	15-30%
T4a	25-30%
T4b	30-40%

Malignant Melanoma of Skin

N Classification
Number of Involved Regional Lymph Nodes

N1	N1a	Single node involved
	N1b	2-4 nodes involved
	N1c	More than 4 nodes involved

Justification. DSK-TNM proposal, different prognosis (Balch et al. [2], Drepper
et al. [8]; Hohenberger et al. [22]).

Size of Involved Regional Lymph Nodes

pN1	pN1 (i)	Only micrometastasis (none larger than 0.2 cm)
	pN1 (ii)	Metastasis to regional lymph nodes, at least one more than 0.2 cm and all $\leq$0.4 cm or less in greatest dimension
	pN1 (iii)	Metastasis to regional lymph nodes, at least one >0.4 cm and all $\leq$3 cm or less in greatest dimension

Justification. Different prognosis (Hermanek [17]; Drepper et al. [8]).

Stage Grouping

A Japanese Group (Yamamoto et al., unpublished data) recommended separating
stage III into

Stage IIIA   pT4   N0   M0   and   Stage IIIB   Any T   N1, N2   M0

An alternative stage grouping is proposed by the German Melanoma Group
(Garbe et al. [11])

Stage I	pT1	N0	M0
Stage II	pT2	N0	M0
	pT3	N0	M0

Both of these stage grouping systems are recommended for testing.

A completely different TNM classification and stage grouping have been proposed by the AJCC*. It cannot be directly compared with the present TNM classification because different criteria for T, N, and M are used. Comparative testing is recommended.

Breast Tumours

T Classification

T1–3   (i)   Without invasion of the underlying fascia and pectoral muscles
        (ii)   With invasion of the underlying fascia and pectoral muscles

Justification. ICC report 1989, for treatment planning.

N Classification

N2   N2a   Nodes fixed to one another
      N2b   Nodes fixed to other structures

Justification. ICC report 1989, for treatment planning.

M Classification

Ml   Mla   Metastasis in supraclavicular lymph nodes (ipsi- and/or contralateral) only
      Mlb   Other distant metastasis

Justification. General considerations, for treatment planning (DSK-TNM).

A proposal for a new stage grouping with a modified N/pN classification and inclusion of grading was published by the AJCC (see reference Yarbro et al., page 117) and is recommended for testing.

Gynaecological Tumours

Cervix Uteri

N Classification

N1   N1a   Metastasis in 1-2 regional lymph nodes below the common iliac artery
      N1b   Metastasis in 3 or more regional lymph nodes below the common iliac artery
      N1c   Metastasis in any lymph node along the common iliac artery

Justification. Dr. Dunst, Erlangen, for treatment planning. Also, data from the literature show the following recurrence rates:

---

* Baloh CHM, Buzaid AC, Atleins MB et al. A new American Joint Committee on Cancer Staffing System for cutaneous melanoma. Cancer 2000; 88: 1484–1491

- pNla, 62% or 81% [1, 42]
- pNlb, 34% or 29% [1, 42]

The 5-year survival was found to be

- 1–3 nodes involved 60% [37]
- 4 or more nodes involved 38% [37]
- pN1 a, b 53% or 63% [24] [27]
- pN1c 21% or 30% [24] [27]

In one investigation [1] the number of involved nodes was found to be an independent prognostic factor by multivariate analysis. The respective classes were 1–2 versus 3 or more nodes involved.

M Classification

M1   M1a   Distant metastasis in paraaortic lymph nodes below the diaphragm only

      M1b   Distant metastasis in other sites

Justification. The 5-year survival rate in patients with para-aortic node metastases only treated by radiotherapy was 29% [35].

Urological Tumours

Penis

T Classification

Tl,T2   a   Tumour 2 cm or lessin greatest dimension

      b   Tumour more than 2 cm but not more than 5 cm in greatest dimension

      c   Tumour more than 5 cm in greatest dimension

Justification. For treatment planning and for comparability with the classification of Maiche and Pyrhönen [30].

Prostate

T Classification

T4a   (i)   Tumour invades bladder neck

      (ii)   Tumour invades external sphincter

      (iii) (i) and (ii)

      (iv) Tumour invades rectum

T4b   (i)   Tumour invades levator muscles

      (ii)   Tumour is fixed to pelvic wall

      (iii) (i) and (ii)

Justification. Insufficient information on prognostic significance, therapeutic implications [41].

M Classification

M1b (i)   Metastasis in bone(s), 1 to 5 foci
      (ii)   Metastasis in bone(s), more than 5, but not more than 20 foci
      (iii) Metastasis in bone(s), more than 20 foci or diffuse metastatic involvement

Justification. Different prognosis [44] recommendation of Schröder et al. [41]. The 2-year survival rates were: M1b(i), 95%; M1b(ii), 75%; M1b(iii), 50% [44].

Kidney

T Classification

T1   T1a Tumour 4.0 cm or less in greatest dimension, limited to the kidney
     T1b Tumour more than 4.0 but not more than 7.0 cm in greatest dimension, limited to the kidney

Justification. Different prognosis according to size [13]; for separate analysis of patients treated by partial nephrectomy.

T1-3a (i)   Without microscopic venous invasion
       (ii) With microscopic venous invasion

Justification. Different prognosis [18, 23].

Ophthalmic Tumours

Retinoblastoma

T Classification

T1   T1a Macula not involved
     T1b Macula involved
T2   T2a Macula not involved
     T2b Macula involved

Justification. Important for evaluation of visual results after treatment [28, 32, 33, 40].

References

[1] Alvarez RD, Soong SJ, Kinney WK, et al. Identification of prognostic factors and risk groups in patients found to have nodal metastasis at the time of radical hysterectomy for early-stage squamous carcinoma of the cervix. *Gynecol Oncol* 1989; **35**: 130–135

[2] Balch CM, Soong SJ, Shaw HM, et al. An analysis of prognostic factors in 8500 patients with cutaneous melanoma. In: *Cutaneous Melanoma* (2nd ed). Balch CM, Houghton AN, Milton GW, Sober AJ, Soong SJ (eds),. Lippincott: Philadelphia, 1992

[3] Breuninger H, Black B, Rassner G. Microstaging of squamous cell carcinoma. *Am J Clin Pathol* 1990; **194**: 624–627

[4] Breuninger H, Langer B, Rassner G. Untersuchungen zur Prognosebestimmung des spinozellulären Karzinoms der Haut und Unterlippe an Hand des TNM-Systems und zusätzlicher Parameter. *Hautarzt* 1988; **39**: 430–434

[5] Bülzebruck H, Hermanek P. Beiträge der Thoraxklinik Heidelberg-Rohrbach zur Weiterentwicklung der TNM-Klassifikation für das Lungenkarzinom. In *20 Jahre Tumortherapie in der Thoraxklinik Heidelberg-Rohrbach der Landesversicherungsanstalt Baden, Rückblick und Ausblick zur Jahrtausendwende.* Drings P, Vogt-Moykopf I (eds) Thoraxklinik Heidelberg-Rohrbach 1999, pp 53–59

[6] Cawthorn SJ, Parums DV, Gibbs NM, et al. Extent of mesorectal spread and involvement of lateral resection margin as prognostic factors after surgery for rectal cancer. *Lancet* 1990; **1**: 1055–1059

[7] Dralle H, Damm I, Scheumann GFW, Kotzerke J, Kupsch E, Geerlings H, Pichlmayr R. Compartment-oriented microdissection of regional lymph nodes in medullary thyroid carcinoma. *World J Surg* 1994; **24**: 112–121

[8] Drepper H, Bieβ B, Hofherr B, et al. The prognosis of patients with stage III melanoma. Prospective long-term study on 286 patients of the Fachklinik Hornheide. *Cancer* 1992; **71**: 1239–1246

[9] Endo M, Takeshita K, Yoshino K. Oesophagoscopy for the diagnosis of superficial oesophageal cancer. *Surg Endosc* 1988; **2**: 205–208

[10] Fielding LP, Arsenault PA, Chapuis PH, et al. Clinicopathological staging for colorectal cancer: An International Documentation System (IDS) and an International Comprehensive Anatomical Terminology (ICAT). *J Gastroenterol Hepatol* 1991; **6**: 325–344

[11] Garbe C, Büttner P, Bertz J, et al. Primary cutaneous melanoma. Identification of prognostic groups and estimation of individual prognosis for 5093 patients. *Cancer* 1995; **75**: 2484–2491

[12] Gelb AG, Sudilovsky D, Wu CD, et al. Appraisal of intratumoral microvessel density, MIB-1 score, DNA content, and p53 protein expression as prognostic indicators in patients with locally confined renal cell carcinoma. *Cancer* 1997; **80**: 1768–1775

[13] Guinan P, Sobin LH, Algaba F, et al. TNM Staging of Renal Cell Carcinoma. Report of Workgroup 3. *Cancer* 1997; **80**: 992–993

[14] Häffner AC, Garbe C, Burg G, et al. The prognosis of primary and metastasising melanoma. An evaluation of the TNM classification in 2495 patients. *Br J Cancer* 1992; **66**: 856–861

[15] Harrison JC, Dean PJ, van der Zwaag R, et al. Adenocarcinoma of the stomach with invasion limited to the muscularis propria. *Hum Pathol* 1991; **22**: 111–117

[16] Hausamen JE. Tasks and objectives of the German-Austrian-Swiss Working Group on Tumours in the Maxillo-Facial Region (DOESAK). *Int J Oral Maxillofac Surg* 1988; **17**: 264–266

[17] Hermanek P. Lymphogene Metastasierung des malignen Melanoms, Häufigkeit, Klassifikation und prognostische Bedeutung. *Acta Chir Austr* 1987; **19**: 249–250

[18] Hermanek P, Schrott KM. Evaluation of the new tumor, nodes and metastasis classification of renal cell carcinoma. *J Urol* 1990; **144**: 238–244

[19] Hermanek P, Hutter RVP, Sobin LH, Wittekind Ch. Classification of isolated tumour cells and micrometastasis. *Cancer* 1999; **86**: 2668–2673

[20] Hermanek P. The superiority of the new International Union Against Cancer and American Joint Committee on Cancer TNM staging of gastric carcinoma. *Cancer* 2000; 88: 1763–1765

[21] Hirayama K, Mori S. Prognostic factors in early esophageal cancer. *Gan To Kagaku Ryoho* 1990; **17**: 37–45

[22] Hohenberger W, Göhl J, Kessler C. Prophylaktische und therapeutische Lymphknotendissektion bei malignem Melanom. *Chirurg* 1993; **32**: 7–9

[23] Höhn W, Hermanek P. Invasion of veins in renal cell carcinoma—frequency, correlation and prognosis. *Eur Urol* 1983; **9**: 276–280

[24] Hsu CT, Cheng YS, Su SC, et al. Prognosis of uterine cervical cancer with extensive lymph node metastases. *Am J Obstet Gynecol* 1972; **114**, 954–962

[25] Inoue K, Tobe T, Kan N, et al. Problems in the definition and treatment of early gastric cancer. *Br J Surg* 1991; **78**: 818–821

[26] Kato H, Tachimori Y, Watanabe H, Iizuka T (1993) Evaluation of the new (1987) TNM classification for thoracic esophageal tumors. *Int J Cancer* 53: 220–223

[27] Kjorstadt KE, Kolbenstvedt A, Strickert T, et al. The value of complete lymphadenectomy in radical treatment of cancer of the cervix, stage IB. *Cancer* 1984; **54**: 2215–2219

[28] Kock E, Rosengren B, Tengroth B, et al. Retinoblastoma treated with a ^{60}Co applicator. *Radiother Oncol* 1986; **7**: 19–26

[29] Krook J, Moertel C, Gunderson LL, et al. Effective surgical adjuvant therapy for high-risk rectal carcinoma. *N Engl J Med* 1991; **324**: 709–715

[30] Maiche AG, Pyrhönen S. Clinical staging of cancer of the penis: by size? by localization? or by depth of infiltration? *Eur Urol* 1990; **18**: 16–22

[31] Marsh JW, Dvorchik I, Bonham CA, Iwatsuki S. Is the pathologic TNM staging system for patients with hepatoma predictive of outcome ? *Cancer* 2000; **88**: 538–543

[32] Migdal C. Bilateral retinoblastoma: the prognosis for vision. *Br J Ophthalmol* 1983; **67**: 592–595

[33] Monge OR, Flage T, Hatlevoll R, et al. Sight-saving therapy in retinoblastoma. Experience with external megavoltage radiotherapy. *Acta Ophthalmol* 1986; **64**: 414–420

[34] Morton DL, Davtyan DG, Wanek LA, et al. Multivariate analysis of the relationship between survival and the microstage of primary melanoma by Clark level and Breslow thickness. *Cancer* 1993; **71**: 3737–3743

[35] Nori D, Valentine E, Hilaris BS, et al. The role of paraaortic node irradiation in the treatment of cancer of the cervix. *Int J Radiat Oncol Biol Phys* 1989; **11**: 1469–1473

[36] Nozaki Y, Yamamoto M, Ikai I, et al. Reconsideration of lymph node metastasis pattern (N Factor) from intrahepatic cholangiocarcinoma using the International Union against Cancer TNM staging system for primary liver carcinoma. *Cancer* 1998; **83**: 1923–1929

[37] Piver MS, Chung WS. Prognostic significance of cervical lesion size and pelvic node metastases in cervical carcinoma. *Obstet Gynecol* 1975; **46**: 507–510

[38] Platz H, Fried R, Hudec M. *Prognoses of oral cavity carcinomas*. Hansen: Munich, 1986

[39] Roder JD, Busch R, Stein HJ, et al. Ratio of involved and removed lymph nodes as a predictor of survival in squamous cell carcinoma of the oesophagus. *Br J Surg* 1994; **81**: 410–413

[40] Schipper J, Tau KEWP, van Peperzeel HA. Treatment of retinoblastoma by precision megavoltage radiation therapy. *Radiother Oncol* 1985; **3**: 97–115

[41] Schröder FH, Hermanek P, Denis L, et al. The TNM classification of prostate cancer. *Prostate* 1992; **Suppl 4**: 129–138

[42] Shiromizu K, Matsuzawa M, Takahashi M, Ishihara O. Is postoperative radiotherapy or maintenance chemotherapy necessary for carcinoma of the uterine cervix? *Br J Obstet Gynaecol* 1985; **195**: 503–506

[43] Siewert JR, Böttcher K, Stein HJ, Roder JD. Relevant prognostic factors in gastric cancer. Ten-year results from the German gastric cancer Study. *Ann Surg* 1998; **228**: 449–461

[44] Soloway MS, Hardeman SW, Hickey DP, et al. Simple grading systems for bone scans correlates with survival for patients with stage D2 prostate cancer. *J Urol* 1987; **137**: 359A

[45] Torres C et al. Pathologic factors in Barrett's associated carcinoma. *Cancer* 1999; **85**: 520–528

[46] Yoshinaka H, Shimazu H, Fukumoto T, Baba M. Superficial esophageal carcinoma: a clinicopathological review of 59 cases. *Am J Gastroenterol* 1991; **86**: 1413–1418

Frequently Asked Questions

General Questions

In Situ Carcinoma

Question
Can one stage in situ carcinoma if the regional lymph nodes have not been assessed, e.g., in a completely resected colonic polyp?

Answer
Although it is strictly NX (Regional lymph nodes cannot be assessed), NX is assumed to be N0 because lymph node metastasis is not consistent with an in situ lesion (see p. 9).

Clinical and Pathological Stage

Question
A patient has a needle biopsy of a left upper lobe mass that is positive for squamous cell carcinoma. A CT of the thorax shows a 4-cm left upper lobe mass >2 cm from the carina. The clinical category is cT2. What is the pathologic classification?

Answer
Biopsy alone is not sufficient for pathological staging in this instance. Resection of the primary tumour is needed for pT1 or pT2 lung tumours to define their limits. Biopsy, without resection, could be used, for example, for pT4 (showing invasion of the oesophagus) (see p. 81).

R Classification

Question
Does R0 mean a complete tumour-free situation or is the R classification limited to the primary?

Answer

R classification is not limited to the primary. The R classification not only considers locoregional residual tumour but also distant residual tumour in the form of unresected or incompletely resected metastases (R2) (see p. 10ff).

R Classification

Question

If there is residual tumour after surgery, is it stage IV?

Answer

RX: Presence of residual tumour can not be assessed.
R0: No residual tumour.
R1: Microscopic residual tumour.
R2: Macroscopic residual tumour.

R2 is not always synonymous with M1 (stage IV) disease. For example, in the absence of distant metastasis (M0), residual macroscopic primary tumour not or incompletely resected by the surgeon is R2.

In another example, a metastasis in the liver from a primary gastric carcinoma would be M1 (Stage IV) and R2 (if the metastasis was not resected). It would be pM1 (stage IV) and R0 if the metastasis was solitary and resected (see p. 10ff).

R Classification and Tis

Question

Lumpectomy specimen of a breast tumour contains a 1.1-cm carcinoma with no invasive carcinoma at the resection lines; however, intraductal carcinoma was at the lateral resection line. How is this classified with respect to T category and R classification?

Answer

The invasive carcinoma would be pT1 and R0. Although the in situ component is not considered in the R classification, an optional solution would be R1(is) (see p. 12).

Positive Cytology

Question

If peritoneal washing cytology, taken before any other procedure during laparotomy is positive, how do I stage the patient ? Grossly visible peritoneal metastases were not found. Is it considered a form of peritoneal metastasis and thus stage IV?

Answer

Positive cytology on lavage of the peritoneal cavity performed during laparoscopy or immediately after opening the abdomen (beginning of laparotomy) corresponds to M1 (except for tumours of corpus uteri, ovary and fallopian tube). Newer data suggest that the worsening of prognosis indicated by positive lavage cytology may have been overestimated. Thus it seems important to analyze such cases separately. For identification of cases with positive cytology from pleural or peritoneal washings as the sole basis for M1, the optional addition of "cy+" is recommended, e.g. M1(cy+) and in the R classification R1(cy+) may be used [1] (see p. 8).

T0 and TX

Question
Explain the difference between TX and T0.

Answer
TX: Primary tumour cannot be assessed.
T0: No evidence of primary tumour.
TX means you were not able to evaluate the tumour, e.g., the extent of a primary testis tumour requires radical orchiectomy; if there is no radical orchiectomy TX is used.
T0 means that a primary tumour was not found by any clinical methods, e.g., if you found a cervical lymph node with metastatic squamous cell carcinoma and you examined the mouth, pharynx, and larynx and found no primary tumour, you would code T0(N1 M0) on the assumption that the primary was in the region (see p. 9).

Synchronous Tumours

Question
What is the rule for classifying a synchronous versus a metachronous second primary tumour?

Answer
If a new primary cancer is diagnosed within two months, the new cancer is considered synchronous; otherwise it is metachronous (based on criteria used by the SEER Program of the National Cancer Institute, USA). Metachronous tumours are classified separately from the preceding tumour. General rule No. 5 (page 3) discusses the rules for classifying simultaneous (synchronous) tumours (see p. 3).

Single Tumour Cells and Micrometastasis in Lymph Nodes

Question
How does one classify single tumor cells detected immunohistochemically in lymph nodes?

Answer

There has been considerable debate in recent years on how to classify tumour cells in lymph nodes or bone marrow that are detected by immunohistochemical or molecular methods. The TNM Project has published an optional proposal to deal with this situation as subsets of N0 (see p. 8).

Single tumour cells should be distinguished from cases with morphologic evidence of micrometastasis, i.e., no metastasis larger than 0.2 cm. The latter can be identified by the addition of (mi) in the pN or pM categories as follows:

pN1 (mi)   Regional lymph node micrometastasis
pM1 (mi)   Distant micrometastasis

(see p. 8).

Number of Lymph Nodes

Question

If less than the desired number of lymph nodes is found, and none shows metastasis, should it be classified as pNX or pN0?

Answer

If the examined lymph nodes are negative, but the number ordinarily resected is not met, classify as pN0. The number of lymph nodes examined and the number involved by tumour should be recorded in the pathology report. This information may be added in parentheses, e.g., for colorectal carcinoma pN0 (0/10) or pN1 (2/11) (see p. 81).

Pathological Assessment of Distant Metastasis

Question

Should liver metastasis diagnosed by fine-needle aspiration (FNA) be considered pM1 or pMX? The primary site is the breast.

Answer

General rule 2 of TNM states, "The pathologic assessment of distant metastasis (pM) entails microscopic examination." This statement intentionally uses the term "microscopic" rather than "histologic" to allow for FNA and cytology. In this case the classification would be pM1 (see p. 2).

Classification of Brain Tumours

Question

The 4th Edition of TNM included a classification for brain tumours. Why has this been left out of the 5th Edition?

Answer
The application of TNM to CNS tumours has not been successful. This particularly concerns the classification as a predictor of outcome. That carries little weight compared with other factors such as histological type, tumour location and patient age. The N does not apply at all, and the M rarely plays a role. This field is still under study to find other means of classifying CNS tumours that will carry prognostic significance.

Classification of Primary Peritoneal Neoplasms

Question
How do you classify primary neoplasms of the peritoneum? We did not find any TNM classification for these tumours. Some of our colleagues use the FIGO/TNM ovary classification.

Answer
Because of the rarity of primary peritoneal neoplasms, there is indeed no TNM classification for them. Basically, there are two primary peritoneal entities: mesothelioma and primary carcinoma of the peritoneum. The latter, serous papillary carcinoma of the peritoneum, according to McCaughey et al. 1986 [3] and Killackey and Davis 1993 [2], has the same prognosis as ovarian tumours. There are no proposals regarding peritoneal mesotheliomas.

Pathological vs. Clinical TNM

Question
Does the pathological TNM replace the clinical TNM?

Answer
No. TNM is a dual system with a (pretreatment) clinical classification (cTNM or TNM) and a (postsurgical histopathological) pathological classification (pTNM). Both classifications are retained unaltered in the patient's record. The former is used for the choice of treatment; the latter is used for the estimation of prognosis and the possible selection of postoperative (adjuvant, additive) therapy (see p. 2).

When in Doubt

Question
If I am not sure of the correct T, N, or M category, e.g., because of unclear measurements, which do I select?

Answer
Select the lower (i.e., less advanced) category.

Example. Sonography of the liver shows a lesion suspicious but not definite for a metastasis. Select M0 (not M1) (see p. 3).

Tumour Cells in Lymphatics

Question

If I have a carcinoma of the colon with invasive tumour in the submucosa, but with lymphatics in the muscularis propria containing tumour cells, which do I select, T1 or T2?

Answer

T1 (submucosa). The microscopic presence of tumour cells in lymph vessels or veins does not qualify as local spread in the T classification (except tumour cells in veins for liver and kidney). The optional L(lymphatic) and V(venous) classifications can be used to record such involvement (see p. 12, 5th ed. TNM Classification).

Tumour Spillage

Question

If tumour is spilled into the abdomen during surgery, how does this affect classification?

Answer

Tumour spillage is considered only in the T classification of ovarian tumours. In the ovary, T1c , rupture of the capsule, includes spontaneous rupture and rupture during surgery. At other sites, it does not affect the TNM or stage grouping (see p. 6).

Simultaneous Tumours

Question

I have a case of a colon with two carcinomas, one invasive into the muscularis propria and the other invasive into the submucosa. How do I code them?

Answer

T2(m) or T2(2). When there are simultaneous (synchronous) tumours in one organ, the tumour with the highest T category is classified and the multiplicity (m) or number of tumours (2) is indicated in parentheses. If bilateral cancers occur simultaneously in paired organs, each tumour is classified independently. For carcinomas of the thyroid, liver, ovary, and fallopian tube multiplicity is a criterion of T classification. If a new primary cancer is diagnosed within 2 months, the new cancer is considered synchronous (criterion of the SEER Program of the NCI, USA) (see p. 3).

Direct Spread

Question

Is a tumour that has spread directly from a gastric primary into an adjacent regional lymph node coded in the T or N category?

Answer
N category. Direct spread into a regional lymph node is classified as lymph node metastasis; direct spread into an adjacent organ, e.g., the liver from a gastric primary, is recorded in the T classification (see p. 9, 5th ed. TNM Classification).

Recurrent Tumour

Question
How can I classify a patient who had an apparently complete local excision of a carcinoma of the rectum, but was found, 2 years later, to have recurrent tumour at the same site?

Answer
Use the Recurrent tumour, r symbol. There must be a documented disease-free interval to use this symbol. For example, rT0N0M0 would designate the status during the disease free interval and rT1N0M0 would indicate a recurrent tumour at the primary site (estimated clinically to be in the submucosa). After a second resection the result might be expressed as: rpT2pN1M0, if the resected tumour was found pathologically to be in the muscularis propria with 2 positive lymph nodes (see p. 12, 5th ed. TNM Classification).

Unknown Primary

Question
How do I classify a patient who has metastatic melanoma in a cervical lymph node <3 cm in greatest dimension without a primary or other metastasis?

Answer
T0N1M0, stage III. The staging is based on regional lymph node and/or distant metastasis status. In this case, the site of metastasis is assumed to be regional (see p. 9).

AJCC vs. UICC TNM

Question
Does the AJCC classification differ from the UICC TNM classification?

Answer
No. The TNM classification in the publications of the UICC and the American Joint Committee on Cancer (AJCC) are identical. They were formulated together, but appear in separate books, namely, the UICC TNM *Classification of Malignant Tumours* and the AJCC *Cancer Staging Manual*. Both are in their fifth editions and were published in 1997.

Sentinel Lymph Node

Question
How do I classify sentinel lymph node status?

Answer
The TNM Committee recommends the following option to record sentinel lymph node status:

- pN0(sn)   No sentinel lymph node metastasis
- pN1(sn)   Sentinel lymph node metastasis
            [5] (see p. 8).

Site-Specific Questions

Larynx

Question
Because the T classification of laryngeal tumours involves assessment of vocal cord fixation, does it mean that pT is not possible without such information given by the clinician?

Answer
For pathological classification concerning impaired mobility or fixation of vocal cords the information from the clinical T is used for the pathologic T. This is in accordance with TNM rule No. 2, pathological classification "is based on the evidence acquired before treatment, supplemented or modified by the additional evidence acquired from surgery and from pathological examination" (see p. 31).

Oesophagus

Question
Is a tumour of the oesophagus with invasion of perioesophageal fatty tissue without infiltration of adjacent structures classified as pT3 or pT4? Does the perioesophageal fatty tissue belong to the mediastinum and thus to adjacent structures?

Answer
pT3. The fatty tissue belongs to the adventitia and not to adjacent structures such as bronchus, heart, pericardial sac and aorta (see p. 33).

Question
For tumours of upper thoracic oesophagus what is the difference between pN1 and pM1a, because the definition of regional lymph nodes of the cervical oesophagus includes supraclavicular lymph nodes?

Answer

For the thoracic oesophagus, including the upper thoracic, the cervical lymph nodes are not regional nodes. For the cervical oesophagus, the regional nodes are the cervical nodes (see p. 34).

Question

If you have an adenocarcinoma of the gastroesophageal junction should you use the TNM classification for an esophageal or gastric primary?

Answer

Gastric tumours located in the cardiac area may involve the distal oesophagus, and primary oesophageal tumours may involve the cardiac area of the stomach. For tumours labeled gastroesophageal, to differentiate between oesophageal and gastric tumours, the following may be considered:

If >50% of the tumour involves the oesophagus, the tumour is classified as oesophageal; if <50%, as gastric.

If the tumour is equally located above and below the oesophagogastric junction or is designated as being at the junction, squamous cell, small cell and undifferentiated carcinomas are classified as oesophageal; adenocarcinomas and signet ring cell carcinomas as gastric.

In the absence of Barrett oesophagus, an adenocarcinoma in both cardia and lower oesophagus is most likely to be gastric (see p. 34).

Colon and Rectum

Question

In carcinoma of the colon is a tumour that has reached the serosal surface classified as pT3 or pT4? What is the definition of reaching the serosa? In some places it is taken to be tumour that is within 1 mm of the serosal surface.

Answer

T3 covers tumours in the subserosa, i.e., those beneath the serosal surface.
T4 applies to tumours that "perforate visceral peritoneum", i.e., the serosal surface (see p. 78).

Question

In adjuvant trials on colorectal carcinomas we make the distinction between T4a and T4b tumours as being the following:

T4a   Invasion of other organs
T4b   Penetration of the serosa

How is the distinction made in the TNM Supplement?

Answer

This distinction applies to tumours of the colon and rectum and is mentioned in this volume as an optional proposal for testing new telescopic ramifications of TNM.

pT4a   Invasion of adjacent organs or structures
pT4b   Perforation of visceral peritoneum (see p. 119).

Question

In a patient with adenocarcinoma of colon there was full-thickness penetration of the wall, 13 positive nodes and also a "free-floating" focus of carcinoma in the peritoneal cavity. No other peritoneal tumour was found Should that be staged as T0, TX or T1?

Answer

The case should be considered M1, because there was tumour in the peritoneal cavity separate from the primary. The primary tumour would be pT3, or if it penetrated the serosa, pT4, and N2 because of the number of nodes involved (see p. 38ff).

Question

Is a rectal carcinoma that extends into the anus a T3 or a T4?

Answer

The TNM Supplement states that: "Intramural direct extension from one subsite (segment) of the colon to an adjacent one is not considered in the T classification. The same applies to intramural direct extension from the rectum to the anal canal". The T category is determined by the depth of penetration (see p. 38).

Question

Is a rectal carcinoma infiltrating the levators to be considered T3 or a T4?

Answer

We suggest coding a rectal carcinoma infiltrating the levators as T4 (invasion of adjacent structures). This is based on

- The poor prognosis
- Difficulty in achieving an R0 state (no residual tumour)
- Radical surgery required

(see p. 38).

Pancreas

Question

Why is involvement of splenic vessels not included in the T4 category of pancreas? If it is not included, is it T3 or is it disregarded and classified solely by size?

Answer

The reason for the formulation was because of surgical treatment. Whereas involvement of splenic vessels does not alter the surgical method (partial or total pancreatectomy includes splenectomy and removal of splenic vessels), in all other situations listed under T4 an extended pancreatectomy with removal of additional adjacent structures is necessary. Involvement of splenic vessels is possible only in tumours that extend directly into the peripancreatic tissue. Thus such tumours are T3 (see p. 42).

Lung

Question
For lung carcinomas, does T2 invasion of visceral pleura mean perforation of pleural membrane?

Answer
T2 invasion of visceral pleura includes either of the following:

- Tumour reaches the elastic membrane of the visceral pleura
- Tumour is present on the surface of the visceral pleura

(see p. 42).

Question
How do I classify a patient with a 2-cm primary adenocarcinoma of the right upper lobe of lung with multiple deposits of adenocarcinoma in the right lower lobe, negative lymph nodes and no other metastasis?

Answer
This is M1 (separate tumour nodules in a different lobe). In case of microscopic confirmation of the tumour nodules it is pM1 (see p. 13).

Question
For clinical staging of lung cancer: Do we need to measure the tumour size on the lung "window" or on the mediastinal "window" of CT scans?

Answer
Perform the measurement on the "window" that is most accurate in your institution. It is presumed that a diagnostic radiologist would be able to indicate which is the most accurate procedure.

Breast

Question
If the clinical T has been determined by physical examination as well as by mammography and ultrasonography, which measurement is used for the cT? For instance: Tumour palpated as 3 cm, mammography shows 2 cm, is it T2 to T1?

Answer
According to a proposal in the TNM Supplement the size for classification in this specific case is: 0.5×3.0 cm $+ 0.5 \times 2.0$ cm $= 2.5$ cm and thus T2 (see p. 46).

Question

Breast carcinoma 2.5 cm in diameter with invasion of the dermis/corium. Is this classified as pT2 or pT4?

Answer

The criteria for classifying a breast tumour T4/pT4 include oedema, peau d'orange or ulceration of the skin of the breast and not invasion of the dermis. The tumour is classified as pT2 (see p. 46).

Question

Infiltrating lobular carcinoma, $3 \times 2 \times 1$ cm, with extensive lymphovascular invasion. Pathology report: dermal lymphatics involved. Should this be classified as T4d (inflammatory carcinoma)? No clinical physical examination data were available.

Answer

Inflammatory carcinoma, T4d, requires the macroscopic (clinical) features to be present. Microscopic involvement of dermal lymphatic vessels alone does not count for classification. Tumour is T2 based on size (see p. 46).

Question

In tumours of the breast, how do we classify invasion of lymphatic vessels in paranodal fatty tissue of the axilla with and without involvement of the axillary lymph nodes?

Answer

Invasion of lymphatic vessels in the axilla is not considered in the TNM classification of breast tumours. The optional L (lymphatic) classification (p. 12, TNM 1997) can be used to describe lymphatic vessel involvement.

Question

How does one classify an isolated tumour nodule in the axillary fat of a patient with breast carcinoma?

Answer

It should be classified as lymph node metastasis (see p. 47).

Question

A 2.3-cm axillary lymph node had a small metastasis of 0.1 cm in greatest dimension. How is that classified, according to the dimensions of the metastasis or to the dimensions of the lymph node?

Answer

The size used for classification is the size of the measured metastasis, not the size of the lymph node that contains the metastasis. The case would be classified as a micrometastasis (≤ 0.2 cm) and coded pN1a (see p. 47).

Question

In a case of Paget disease of the nipple with a small 0.3 cm tumour of the breast near the nipple, is this classified as pT1a or pT4?

Answer
This is classified pT1a. Paget disease associated with a tumour is classified according to the size of the tumour (p. 125, TNM 1997).

Question
How is microinvasive (≤1 mm) breast cancer coded in the TNM?

Answer
It is coded as T1mic or pT1mic and is staged the same way as T1 (see p. 125, TNM 1997).

Question
How does one classify breast cancer after chemotherapy? Is pTpN appropriate?

Answer
"In those cases in which classification is performed during or following initial multimodality therapy, the TNM or pTNM categories are identified by a y prefix" (TNM Classification 1997, p. 11). For example, yT1N0M0 or ypT1pN0M0.

Question
The 1997 TNM Classification of breast tumours states: The clinical T1 category is further subclassified into T1mic, T1a, T1b, T1c. There was a discussion among physicians here as to why this was included in the clinical description, because microscopic invasion can only be defined pathologically.

Answer
Histologic examination is required on all clinical classifications for "confirmation of the disease". Pathologic classification, pT, requires more than histologic examination. It "requires the examination of the primary tumour with no gross tumour at the margins of resection" (see p. 127, TNM 1997).

Question
What is the pT category and the R status of a 1.5 cm breast carcinoma detected histologically in the resection margin?

Answer
The pT category is pT1c and the R status R1 (see pp. 13, 125, TNM 1997).

Question
How does one classify a breast tumour with invasion of the nipple/mammilla with or without ulceration?

Answer
The nipple is not considered in the definitions of the T classification. Size and ulceration are relevant criteria for the T category.

Example. Breast carcinoma 1.9 cm in diameter with invasion of the nipple

With ulceration of the nipple   T4b/pT4b
Without ulceration of the nipple   T1c/pT1c

(see p. 126, TNM 1997).

Question
How do we classify a lymph node metastasis of breast cancer with a size of 1.8 mm and extension beyond the lymph node capsule?

Answer
It should be classified as pN1biii, on the basis of extension beyond the capsule and size (See p. 128, TNM 5th edition).

Corpus Uteri

Question
A uterine corpus tumour extends into the parametrium. Should it be classified as T2 or T3a?

Answer
T3a. T2 tumours invade the cervix but do not extend beyond the uterus (see p. 148, TNM 1997).

Question
A radical hysterectomy specimen shows an adenocarcinoma penetrating the serosal surface (pT3a) of the corpus uteri. All regional lymph nodes were negative, but there was metastatic adenocarcinoma in parametrial soft tissue. Does this change the stage of the tumour?

Answer
T3a includes "discontinuous involvement of adnexa and serosa within the pelvis" (see p. 148, TNM 1997).

Prostate

Question
During a radical prostatectomy for transitional cell carcinoma, if we find a clinically unexpected bilateral prostatic adenocarcinoma, should we consider it as incidental (pT1) or as a pT2 tumour?

Answer
There is no pT1 category, therefore pT2 (see p. 172, TNM 1997).

Kidney

Question
We resected a renal cell carcinoma. Histology showed a small focus of tumour in the peripelvic fat and tumour invasion into blood vessels. What would be the T category?

Answer
Invasion of the peripelvic fat would place this case into pT3a category. Histologic identification of blood vessel involvement does not justify pT3b because
this specifically requires grossly visible invasion (see p. 181, TNM 1997).

Question
In the TNM for renal cell carcinoma, a tumour which involves the adrenal
gland is stated as T3. It is not stated, however, whether this is referring to the
ipsilateral kidney. Is spread to the contralateral kidney M1?

Answer
Spread to the contralateral adrenal gland as well as to contralateral kidney is
M1 (see p. 54).

Bladder

Question
For carcinoma of the bladder, if there is involvement of the seminal vesicle,
should it be regarded as pT4a?

Answer
If the wall of the seminal vesicle or stroma of the prostate are involved, it should
be T4a. If there is only in situ carcinoma in the seminal vesicle, it should not be
classified T4. There are data that CIS in the prostatic ducts does not adversely
impact survival [4] (see p. 56).

References

[1] Hermanek P, Hutter RVP, Sobin LH, Wittekind Ch. Classification of isolated
    (disseminated, circulating) tumour cells and micrometastasis. *Cancer* 1999;
    86: 2668–2673
[2] Killackey MA, Davies AR. Papillary serous carcinoma of the peritoneal
    surface: matched-case comparison with papillary serous ovarian carcinoma.
    Gynecol Oncol 1993; **51**: 171–174
[3] McCaughey WT, Schryer MJ, Lin X, et al. Extraovarian pelvic serous
    tumour with marked calcification. *Arch Pathol Lab Med* 1986; **110**: 78–80
[4] Montie JE, Wojno K, Klein E, et al. Transitional cell carcinoma in situ of
    the seminal vesicles: 8 cases with discussion of pathogenesis, and clinical
    and biological implications. *J Urol* 1997; **158**: 1895–1898
[5] Sobin LH. Frequently asked questions regarding the application of the TNM
    classification. *Cancer* 1999; **85**: 1405–1406